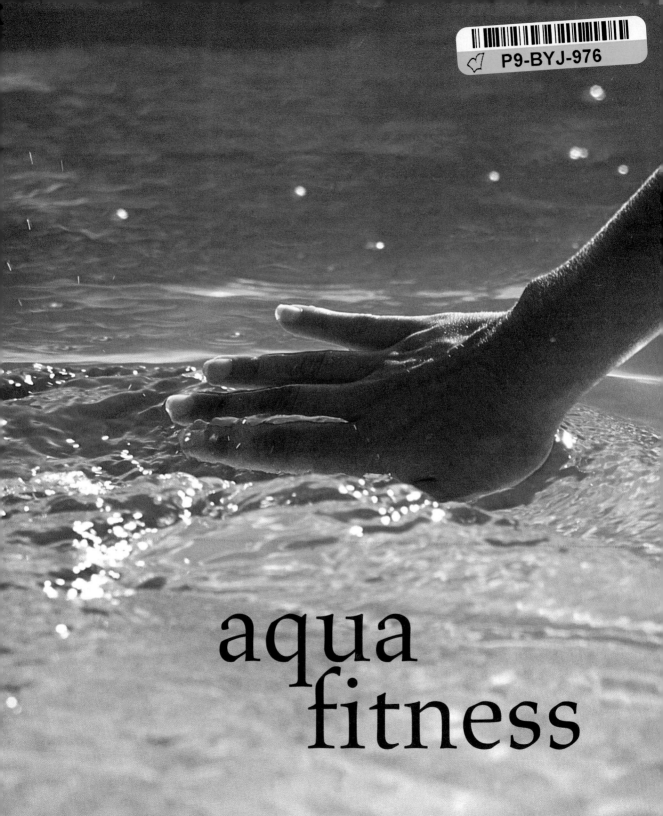

aqua
fitness

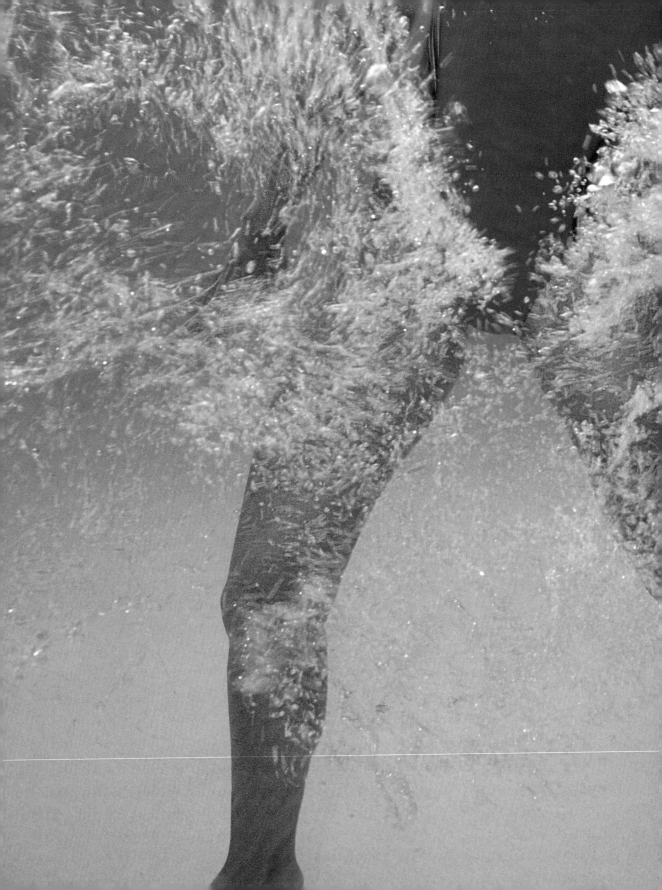

MIMI RODRIGUEZ ADAMI

aqua
fitness

The low-impact total body

fitness workout

DK Publishing

DK

LONDON, NEW YORK, MUNICH, MELBOURNE, and DELHI

Project Editor Irene Lyford
Art Editor Miranda Harvey
Senior Editor Jennifer Jones
Managing Editor Gillian Roberts
Category Publisher Mary-Clare Jerram
Art Director Tracy Killick
DTP Designer Sonia Charbonnier
Production Controller Louise Daly

First American edition, 2002
02 03 04 05 10 9 8 7 6 5 4 3 2 1

Published in the United States by
DK Publishing, Inc.
375 Hudson Street
New York, NY 10014

ISBN 0-7894-8949-X

Color reproduced in Singapore by Colourscan
Printed and bound in Germany by MOHN media and
Mohndruck GmbH

See our complete product line at
www.dk.com

CONTENTS

INTRODUCTION TO
AQUA
FITNESS

Movement, water, and music — three elements that are basic to life. The body needs movement to maintain health and well-being; it needs water to sustain its most essential functions; and music ... well, music is the most universal of languages, giving us joy and comfort, and providing us with a motivation and stimulus to exercise or to relax. Aquafitness is a combination of these three elements that are so fundamental to our lives. Turn the pages and enter a fresh, new world.

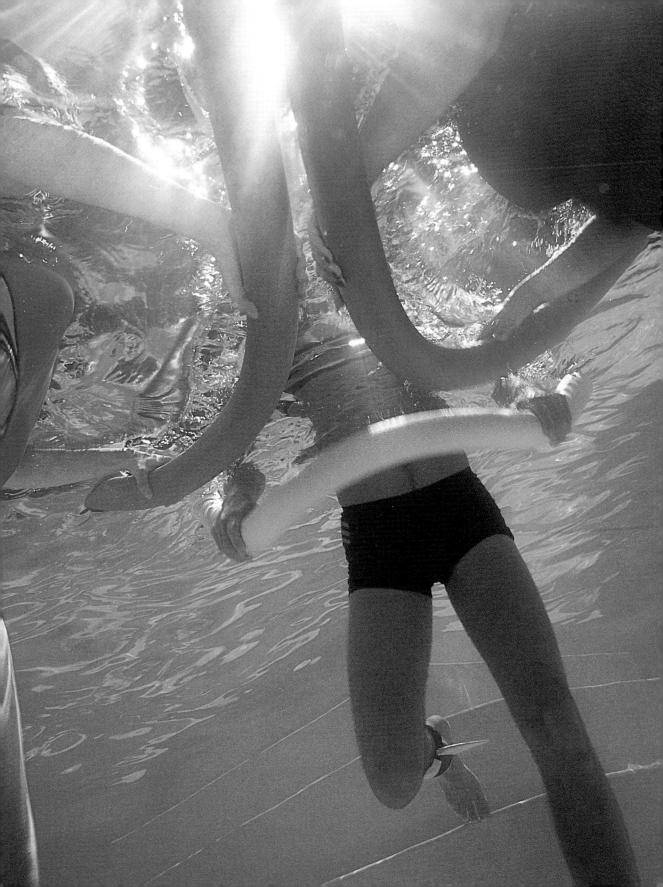

WHAT IS AQUAFITNESS?

This immensely enjoyable form of exercise makes creative use of the natural resistance and buoyancy of water to provide a low-impact workout that is both fun and effective. It is suitable for all ages and different levels of fitness. Aquafitness workouts aim to improve all the components of fitness: muscular endurance and strength, body composition, aerobic capacity, and flexibility or joint mobility, as well as improving neuromuscular coordination.

I have always loved the water. My mother still recounts how hard it was to get me out of the bathtub when I was a toddler. She also tells of my love for music and how, whenever I heard music, I would dance. Music is a very special energy that permeates every cell of my body and produces movement, in one form or another.

When aerobics arrived on the scene in the early 80s, my immediate reaction was: "They've invented this for me!" In fact, I firmly believe that the fitness movement is part of my life journey. In 1988, I tried putting exercise to music in the water and loved it. In Rome, Italy, where I live and work, however, it was still too early. In 1995 I tried again, and then the time was right. I became certified by the Aquatic Exercise Association and brought their program to Italy for other fitness instructors interested in water fitness. In translating all the documentation from English to Italian I had to think of a name for this training modality and came up with "aquafitness" — because this method is more than aerobics: it trains the whole being, in its entirety.

I love what I do: I love teaching class for the wonderful people who work out with me, as well as passing on my knowledge to new generations of aquafitness instructors. And I have loved writing this book, sharing with you my love of water, movement, and music. In the book I have simplified technical language in order to reach a wider audience. But no matter where you live, as long as you have water that reaches your ribs and you can sing a song, the joy of aquafitness is within your reach.

BENEFITS OF AQUAFITNESS

• Provides a low-impact workout that will not strain the weight-bearing joints or the back.

• The resistance of water ensures that the exerciser does not work beyond his or her capability.

• The working heart rate in water is lower than when training at a similar intensity on land.

• Increases or at least maintains bone density.

• Works muscles that are rarely used on land and are consequently flabby.

• Forces the exerciser to maintain abdominal stability during all movements in the water.

• Hydrostatic pressure (the pressure of water on the body) improves blood circulation and helps decrease water retention.

• There is no next-day muscle pain after a workout, but you will sleep really well that night.

• Even though you perspire during the workout, you will never feel sweaty.

• Water exercise is healthy and in vogue .

• The exerciser is "hidden" by the water, which can appeal to those lacking in self-confidence.

• You don't need to know how to swim.

• You don't have to get your hair wet.

• It's fun!

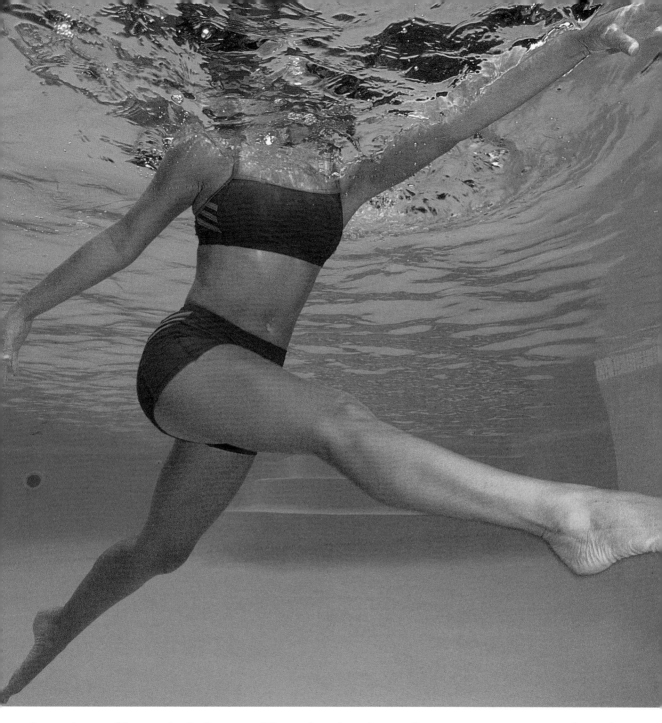

Improving aerobic capacity, body composition, and flexibility. The larger the movements performed during a workout, the more oxygen has to be transported to the muscles in order to generate the energy required to perform the exercise. This trains the cardiorespiratory system and results in a more effective aerobic capacity, which will improve your overall fitness. Working against the resistance of water requires a greater expenditure of energy (and calories) than land-based exercises, which is good news for those seeking to lose weight. At the same time, the large range of movements required to improve muscular endurance and aerobic capacity promotes muscle flexibility and joint mobility. In our workouts, we will always try to work in a full range of motion.

CHARACTERISTICS OF WATER

We're used to moving around on land — it's our natural environment. Moving in water is very different, and it is worth taking a moment to try to understand this familiar yet very different experience. Water has several characteristics in common with air; the difference is that water is 800 times more dense than air, so the effects of those qualities are more pronounced.

Viscosity

This is the friction that occurs between molecules, causing them to stick to each other. It is felt much more in water than on land, and is responsible for the resistance our bodies experience when we try to move in water. It also accounts for the adhesion of the water molecule to anything immersed in it. This phenomenon is illustrated by what happens when you execute a movement in water, then stop. Initially, the water is still, but it then accompanies the body in its movement. When the body stops moving, however, the water continues its motion.

Drag

This term refers to the resistance experienced by a body when moving through water, due to its viscosity. Drag resistance is found in opposition to any movement performed in the water. It is, therefore, a major factor in determining the intensity of your workout.

Turbulence

Whenever you move through water, it reacts by creating waves, eddies, and whirlpools. The more movement performed, the more turbulence results. This disturbance of the water's stillness also increases the muscular effort necessary to move through the water. Consider two examples: the first is walking through still water, such as in a swimming pool; the second is walking through water at the beach, at the point where the waves are breaking. You will agree that the latter situation requires a great deal more exertion.

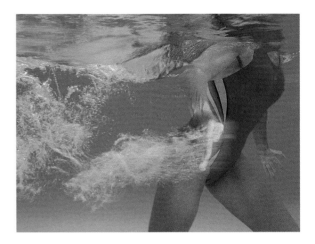

Moving your hand through the water will create eddies and turbulence, which, in turn, will increase the workload of any body trying to pass through them.

Frontal surface area

This refers to the part of the body that is pushing against the water's resistance as it moves. The larger the frontal surface area, the more difficult it is to move against the water's resistance. For example, if you want to move your arm through the water creating as little resistance as possible, hold your hand flat and slice it through the water. If, on the other hand, you want to increase the difficulty of the movement, hold your hand open so that the palm or the back of the hand faces the water as it travels. The greater the frontal surface area, the more the intensity will increase.

Lever length

The question of lever length affects hand and foot positions and the length of limb chosen to perform an exercise. To make an exercise easier you will shorten the limb. For example, crossing bent arms (short lever) in front of the body instead of straight arms (long lever) will notably decrease the intensity of the movement. Another example: a straight leg kick (long lever) is much more difficult to perform repeatedly than a knee lift (short lever). Lengthening the limb increases the frontal surface area and the load on the joint.

THE EFFECTS OF BUOYANCY

When exercising on land, we increase or decrease the intensity of a workout by altering the rate at which we are moving. When working in water, however, we use the properties of water to modify intensity, using the water as if it were equipment.

Anything that has a specific density lower than that of the water itself will be pushed vertically upward. This vertical force is called buoyancy and it works in exactly the opposite way of the force of gravity (the vertical force that attracts all objects toward the center of the Earth.) The deeper the water, the greater the extent to which buoyancy overrides gravity. This has a profound effect on our attempts to exercise in water.

On land, raising your leg in a "high kick" is difficult because you have to lift the weight of your leg against the force of gravity; the higher you kick, the harder it is. A high kick in water, however, is easy to perform. The buoyancy of the water, aided by the fatty tissue in the leg (fat floats because it's less dense than water), helps the muscle pull the leg up toward the water's surface. On the other hand, pulling the leg back down through the water will be much more difficult because you then have to overcome buoyancy to force the leg back down. In aquafitness exercises, you will find that while the primary resistance in water comes from the drag forces of water resistance, you will also be using muscle groups that you normally don't use on land in order to overcome the water's buoyancy.

As well as making certain movements easier, buoyancy has one very pleasing effect for older people. After a certain age, excess flesh tends to droop, due to the force of gravity. In the water, however, all my older clients savor the uplifting effects of buoyancy, even if they are only temporary!

When working out in the water you will find that the water's drag properties and buoyancy make the exercise experience different from that on land. Movement in any direction will be against the water's resistance and you will have to use muscles that are normally passive on land, where gravity aids their common movements. Moving against the multidirectional resistance of water works all the muscles and helps promote muscle balance. In aquafitness, every muscle has to work.

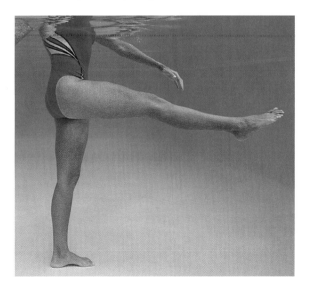

Short lever A kneelift is a short lever movement. The frontal surface area is minimal, so the intensity required for the movement's execution is also minimized.

Long lever A high kick is a long lever movement and, as such, has an increased frontal surface area. It is therefore considered a high intensity movement.

WHAT IS FITNESS?

According to the European Network of Fitness Associations (ENFA), "Fitness is a dynamic state of physical, psychological, and social well-being, as promoted by activity, adapted to individual competence, possibilities, and needs/preferences of persons who take responsibility for their own functioning." Being fit means making the most of being alive. Movement is vital: the more active a person is, the more active he or she is capable of being.

FIVE COMPONENTS OF FITNESS

There are five conditions that must be satisfied in order to attain complete fitness. All are of equal importance and, for true fitness, they must be in balance.

Aerobic capacity

Otherwise described as cardiorespiratory fitness, this refers to the capacity of the cardiovascular and respiratory systems to deliver oxygen to the working muscles for sustained periods of energy production. According to the American College of Sports Medicine (ACSM), to increase or maintain aerobic capacity you must dedicate at least 20 minutes per day on at least three days each week to some type of physical activity that uses the large muscle groups rhythmically and continuously in a complete range of motion. More energy and oxygen are required, the heart becomes stronger, the circulatory system becomes more efficient, cardiorespiratory endurance increases – and you will be able to do more, for longer, without tiring.

Muscular strength

This refers to the maximum force that can be generated by a muscle or muscle group against a resistance. It is an important part of fitness, but the achievement of maximum muscle strength requires the use of heavy weights, or working out with heavy loads on weight-room machines. It would be hard to achieve comparable results without such equipment, but you can certainly improve muscle strength levels by training in water.

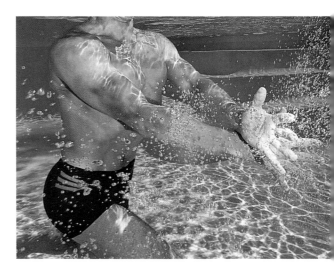

In aquafitness you will train all five fitness components in each workout and experience the benefits of improved endurance, muscle tone, and body composition.

Muscular endurance

This is the ability to continue physical activity, resisting muscular fatigue. It determines how many times you can repeat an action before fatigue forces you to stop; or how long you can hold a position before the muscles tire. Muscular endurance and cardiovascular endurance are closely related and it is important to increase both proportionately because, without aerobic endurance, you will not be able to increase your muscle endurance, and vice versa. By increasing muscle endurance you will indirectly be increasing your muscle strength as well, since the more your muscles resist succumbing to fatigue, the stronger they will be overall. To maintain muscle mass, the ACSM recommends at least 2–3 workouts per week, including at least one set of 8–12 repetitions of a full range of motion muscle contraction for each of the body's 8–10 major muscle groups.

Flexibility / joint mobility

Muscular flexibility is the muscle's ability to safely stretch to its maximum capacity. Joint mobility is the ability to move a body part around the joint in a full range of motion. This is probably the least considered of the fitness components, yet strength and flexibility are closely linked and imbalance can result in injury. The ACSM recommends stretching each major muscle group statically and dynamically at least 2–3 times per week.

Body composition

This refers to the ratio between lean tissue and fatty tissue in the body. Lean tissue (or fat-free mass) includes muscle, bones, organs, and connective tissue. You probably know what fatty tissue is – but it is important to know that a certain amount of fat is indispensable to survival. Essential body fat amounts to about 5 percent of total body mass in men and up to 15 percent in women. When you exercise, you are ultimately training to modify your body composition. Working on your muscle strength and endurance will increase your lean tissue mass, while working on your aerobic capacity will enhance your fat utilization, resulting, hopefully, in an optimal proportion between lean and fatty tissue.

According to the Aerobics and Fitness Association of America (AFAA), the ideal percentage of body fat in men is 12–17 percent and in women 18–22 percent.

While these numbers give an objective measure, the important thing is your health – how you feel, how much energy you have, and how much endurance you have to do more and to get the most out of life.

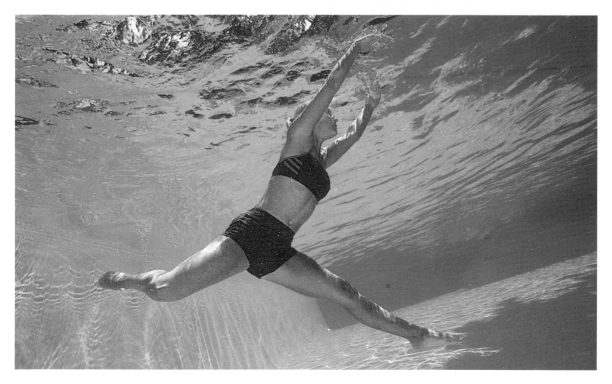

Aquafitness workouts enhance flexibility by allowing you to perform and repeat movements that would be beyond many people's capability on land.

MUSCLES AND MOVEMENT

In starting an exercise program, it is useful to know where muscles are located and how they work. An important fact about muscle tissue is that the more you train it, the more toned it will be. But if you stop exercising you will lose the tone. Use it or lose it!

Muscle contractions

When you initiate a movement, a message is sent from the brain via the nervous system to each individual muscle cell that must be stimulated. Muscles contract in different ways but, in aquafitness, we will be dealing mainly with two types – isometric and isotonic.

In an **isometric contraction**, tension is developed in the muscle, though there is no movement. For example, we use isometric contractions to hold a tray out in front of us. The biceps muscle is flexed but the arm does not move. The tension in the muscle is constant.

The **isotonic contraction** is of particular interest in exercise. The muscle can either shorten or lengthen, causing the movement of the two bones to which it is attached. In a **concentric isotonic** (or positive) **contraction** the muscle shortens. Because of resistance, all movements in water result in concentric contractions.

In an **eccentric isotonic contraction**, the muscle lengthens to sustain a resistance, but is overcome by it. For example, if you are holding a weight with your arm out to the side, eventually the weight is more than you can hold. To avoid hurting yourself, you control the descent of the arm, holding the weight against the force of gravity. This is an eccentric isotonic contraction. In water, such a contraction does not occur unless buoyancy equipment is used. For this reason, water exercise rarely causes day-after pain, which is usually caused by performing eccentric contractions.

Muscle relationships

Muscles usually work in pairs, both muscles crossing the same joint but on different sides. Examples include the biceps and triceps in the upper body; the abdominals

MUSCLE GLOSSARY

Abductor Pulls the leg away from the body's midline.

Adductor Pulls the leg in toward the body's midline.

Anterior tibialis Pulls the foot upward, as when walking or running.

Biceps Responsible for bending the arms and moving the hand toward the face.

Deltoids (Delts) Used in any shoulder movements, such as raising the arms.

Erector spinae Responsible for the backward movement of the spine.

Gastrocnemius and soleus The calf muscles, used in pushing the forefoot down and for pointing the toe.

Gluteus maximus (Glutes) Pulls the leg back or pushes the leg down or turns it out.

Hamstrings A group of three muscles on the back of the thigh that bend the knee, bringing the foot up behind the glutes.

Latissimus dorsi (Lats) Responsible for lowering the arms toward the body or pulling the arms down and behind the body.

Oblique abdominals (Obliques) Responsible for any twisting or side-bending movements.

Pectoralis major (Pecs) Used to move the arms in front and across the body.

Quadriceps (Quads) Used to straighten the leg.

Rectus abdominus Stimulates forward bending of the spine and the pelvic tilt.

Rhomboid Pulls the shoulder blades in toward each other.

Triceps Allow you to straighten your arms in pushing movements.

Trapezius (Traps) Pulls the shoulder blades down and back toward each other. Also used to shrug the shoulders.

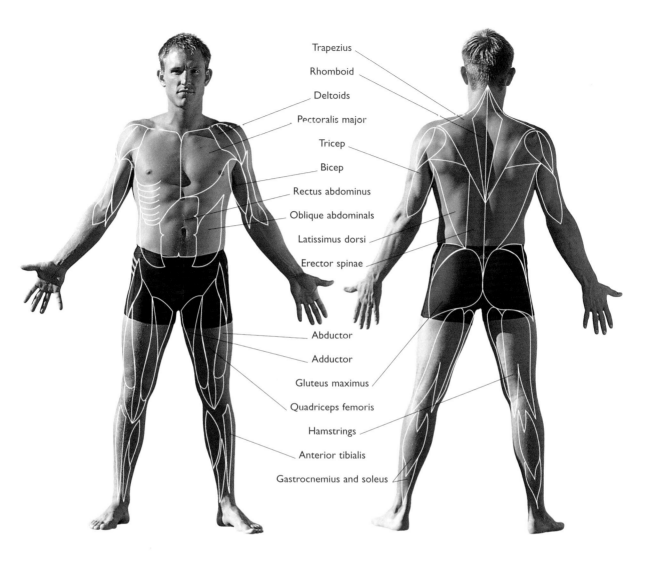

Trapezius

Rhomboid

Deltoids

Pectoralis major

Tricep

Bicep

Rectus abdominus

Oblique abdominals

Latissimus dorsi

Erector spinae

Abductor

Adductor

Gluteus maximus

Quadriceps femoris

Hamstrings

Anterior tibialis

Gastrocnemius and soleus

Anterior muscles usually act as pushers. We tend to work more on the anterior part of the body because it is what we see.

and the erector spinae in the center, and the quadriceps and hamstrings in the lower body. All exercises will be presented using opposing muscle groups.

Stabilizing positions in muscle-conditioning
When you exercise solely to improve muscle tone, you will need to isolate muscles so that most of the energy expended will go to performing the relevant isotonic

Posterior muscles usually act as pullers. It is important to maintain muscle balance, working both front and back muscles proportionately to avoid injury.

contractions. To do this you must stabilize your core muscles (that is the abdominal and erector spinae muscles) against the action/reaction forces created by the movements of the arms and legs. Your core muscles will be constantly engaged in stabilizing your trunk, but without using the energy that should be used in performing the particular exercises. See the stabilizing positions on p23.

NEUROLOGICAL COMPONENTS

We've already looked at some of the major elements of fitness, including cardiovascular (or aerobic) endurance and muscle strength and endurance. Now we turn to motor skills — an area governed by the body's neurological system — and in particular the coordinative capabilities that allow the individual to learn, organize, control, and transform movement.

Balance, agility, and orientation

Balance refers to the body's ability to control and maintain its position against an outside force, or the force of gravity, or — in the water — buoyancy. Static or dynamic, it is based on information received from the neuromuscular system and the senses, particularly vision.

Agility is based on maintaining balance, and refers to the body's ability to move quickly in various directions while maintaining a stable center of gravity.

Orientation is a skill that is based on both balance and agility. It refers to the body's ability to maintain balance while modifying its position in relation to itself, to objects, and to other forces. For example, you are walking up a hill and face right to talk to a friend, while handing a large package with both hands to another person on your left. If a strong gust of wind hits you from the front and you manage to complete your movements without losing balance, then it's safe to say that your orientation capability is good.

Combining motor skills

Most of us are familiar with the subway, metro, or underground. In order to enter the platform you must put a coin or ticket in a slot, which allows you go through a turnstile. This involves a number of different, separate activities that must be coordinated if the process is to be performed as smoothly as possible: modifying your speed and stride length as you approach the turnstile, correctly aiming the coin or ticket at the slot, judging the time necessary to register the payment before pushing the turnstile, speeding up

your pace once you're through so you can make that train, and so on. Now think about coordinating the same series of movements with a shopping bag in your "free hand." Combining motor skills can be quite a feat.

Time–space differentiation

This refers to the ability to estimate the time required to perform a task in a chosen way. The task is analyzed, evaluated, and broken down into simple processes on the basis of the time needed to perform each action. Evaluation continues as the task is performed and any deviations from the predicted rate are integrated in order to complete the activity in the predetermined time. Let's say you are in your car, approaching a red light that is about to change to green. There are no cars in the lane ahead, or crossing the junction. If you have good time–space differentiation skills, you will decrease your speed as you approach the traffic light so that you can accelerate away as soon as it changes to green. You have assessed the distance to be covered and the time needed to cover that distance, modifying the speed of the vehicle in order to avoid coming to a complete stop.

Dynamic differentiation

We have already seen what happens when we go through a subway turnstile, or approach traffic lights. Now it's time to look at more complex behavior, such as skiing, which requires even more complicated neurological fitness. Imagine you're coming down a ski-run, along with numerous other skiers and snow-boarders. Your objective is to get safely down to the ski lodge, without causing any damage to yourself or others. You speed up and slow down on the basis of other skiers' movements and you aim to go around the moguls (bumps) and between the icy patches. Dynamic differentiation refers to the ability of individuals to discern, differentiate, and analyze sensations received through the senses from various objects and events; the knowledge thus gained is then used to respond to further needs, stemming from other activities.

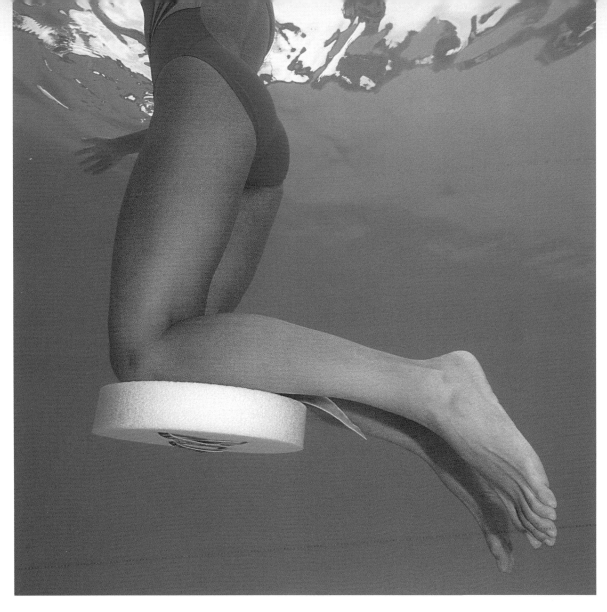

Motor anticipation

You're still skiing; someone falls in the gap between two icy patches that you were aiming for, and you're going too fast to stop. If you hit the other skiier, you will both be hurt; if you fall, you'll slide into the other skier, again causing injury. If you turn quickly, you will avoid him or her and maybe hit the icy patch, but in that case you can flatten out your skis and glide over it, braking when you hit the snow on the other side. What do you do? Motor anticipation is the ability to assess and predict the outcome of an action and program a subsequent activity on the basis of that forecast.

Balance is the most basic part of coordination because it is intrinsic to all the other capabilities. Training for balance in water is both effective and safe.

Movement creativity

This refers to the ability to continuously create original and creative forms of movement and infinite variations of them. These make up your movement library: they are how you express yourself through movement, and are based on your particular body proportions, the sports or disciplines that you have practiced during your lifetime, and the type of music that you like.

EXERCISE PRINCIPLES

Many principles are involved when developing a fitness program. Understanding these will help you to work out safely and effectively and to obtain positive results from your efforts. While some may try to convince you that a strong, healthy, fit body can be obtained effortlessly, this is not true. However, a regular exercise program of moderate intensity will ensure your well-being and enhance your self-esteem and quality of life.

EXERCISE TERMINOLOGY

Certain terms crop up regularly in exercise manuals and fitness classes. Understanding these will help you to appreciate the theoretical basis on which fitness programs are constructed, and to apply that knowledge to your own fitness program.

Adaptation refers to biochemical, structural, mechanical, and/or physiological modifications that make it easier for the body to perform the same action in the future. Also known as the training effect, it includes the benefits that result from any activity undertaken.

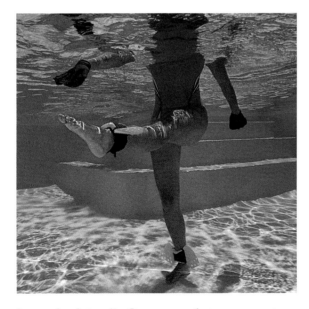

Increasing intensity Once you perfect a movement, step up the intensity by using equipment. Here, aquafins make the hip flexors work harder during high kicks.

Initial response This principle states that those who have the worst initial capabilities have the best chance of improving their condition. The more you have to gain, the more you can gain; conversely, the more you have to lose, the more you can lose.

Intensity is a measure of the stress or demand placed upon a physiological system during the training activity.

Overload forms the basis for any training program. A greater than normal stress or demand placed upon a physiological system or organ typically results in an increase in strength or function.

Progressive overload refers to a gradual and systematic increase in the stress or demand placed upon a physiological system in order to cause an adaptation without risking chronic fatigue or injury.

Reversibility This principle is probably the most depressing aspect of any exercise program, but one that needs to be understood. It states that the body will gradually return to the state it was in at the start of the exercise program if the individual stops exercising. It emphasizes the need for regular, continuous exercise.

Specificity is the principle that states that adaptation occurs only in that part of the organism that is being stimulated or overloaded.

Variability This principle, which underlies cross-training, states that in order to obtain better muscle balance and overall fitness, it is necessary to vary the intensity, the duration, or the way a workout is performed. In other words, you have to exercise in different ways in order to stimulate a change in different aspects of your body.

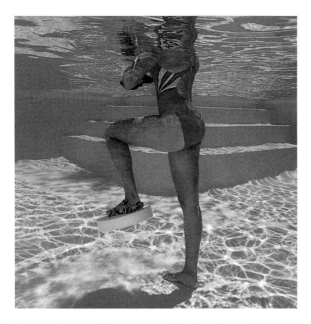

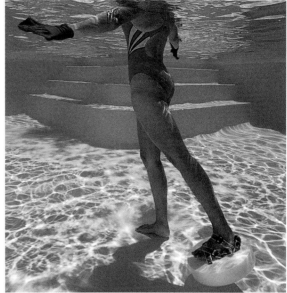

Variability A closed chain disk and webbed gloves are being used here in order to vary the way in which the various muscle groups are being stimulated.

Action/Reaction By pushing the arms and leg back, the body will be propelled forward. But if you push the arms forward you will contrast this.

THE LAWS OF MOTION

The fundamental principles of exercise are based on Isaac Newton's three laws of motion. These operate on land as well as in water, but their effects are noticeably more pronounced in water. The aim of most workouts is to increase fitness level and burn calories. An understanding of Newton's laws will help you to make the most of your aquafitness workout by modifying your energy expenditure and your oxygen consumption.

Inertia Newton's first law states that an object remains at rest or in a state of uniform motion unless acted upon by an outside force. This refers to the energy needed to move an object from rest and to stop an object that is in motion. The more you move, the more energy you'll expend, so the exercise will be more intense and you'll burn more calories. You start by just moving your legs, then you add your arms (limb inertia), then you start traveling in the water (body inertia), and finally you change direction in the water to work against the water's inertia.

Acceleration Put simply, this law states that the harder you push something, the more it will move, and the larger or heavier it is, the harder you have to push it to make it move. It has nothing to do with speed. If performing an exercise in a certain range of motion is too difficult, then by decreasing the range of motion — for example by taking smaller steps — you will also be decreasing the effort needed to perform it.

Action/Reaction For every action there is an equal and opposite reaction. If you want to walk forward in the water, you will have to push the water backward with your hands and arms. This is so natural that you don't even have to think about it. By pushing the water backward, the reaction will be propelling the body forward. If you want to increase the intensity, then you can push the water forward as you move forward through the water — that is really hard. This holds true of any movement and in any direction. If you want to go backward, for example, you will facilitate the movement by kicking forward, and vice versa.

HOW TO EVALUATE INTENSITY

Intensity is the amount of energy you expend in terms of strength, endurance, or flexibility in order to execute a chosen exercise. If you create a greater than normal intensity level, you will induce your body to become more fit. However, working at too high an intensity level can cause fatigue, muscle soreness, or injury. You need to increase intensity progressively and gradually.

Muscular intensity

We have already discussed the importance of overload to adaptation or improved fitness. On land, muscle overload usually means using weights, which, in water, would not be appropriate. Instead, we have to think in terms of drag, inertia, acceleration, action/reaction, lever lengths, frontal surface area, turbulence, as well as the use of specialized aquafitness equipment.

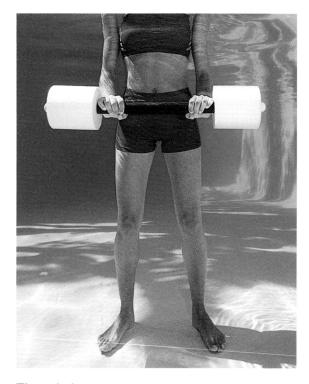

The swimbar increases intensity in two ways; you must overcome buoyancy to keep it under water, and over-come drag forces to push it back and forth in the water.

Let us look at how water can be used as if it were equipment in order to increase the workload on the exercising muscles and the stabilizing muscles.

Buoyancy vs. Gravity

In water, buoyancy is the force that you must overcome in order to keep your feet on the ground and your arms by your sides. The deeper the water, the harder you must work. Just as we use weights on land to overload our muscles and make us stronger, so, in the water, we use buoyancy equipment of differing densities. These require varying degrees of strength to overcome the buoyancy and keep the object submerged. The intensity of the muscle contractions in both pushing the object down and controlling its return to the surface will depend upon the density of the buoyant material, the depth of the water, and the subcutaneous fatty tissue of the exerciser. The more buoyant the equipment and the exerciser, and the deeper the water, the more difficult it will be to push the equipment down, to maintain contact with the floor, and to stabilize the core muscles.

Levers/frontal surface area

There are two other options in modifying muscular intensity in the water. By working with straight arms and legs (long lever) you'll be working harder than if you work out using bent arms and legs (short lever). This is because the longer lever length feels as if it weighs more with respect to the joint. At the same time, the surface area presented to the water during the movement of the straight arm or leg is greater than that presented with a short lever. So, what does that mean in practical terms? If you want to increase the intensity of a knee lift, do a straight leg kick instead. Or, if you want to decrease the intensity on the shoulder joint of an arm sweep, bend the elbow. This concept includes hand and feet positions. If you want to increase intensity, put your extended hand flat to the direction of the movement; if you want to

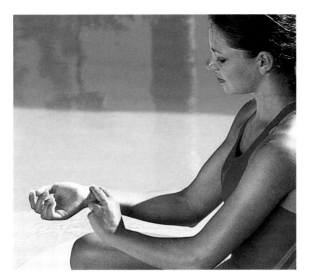

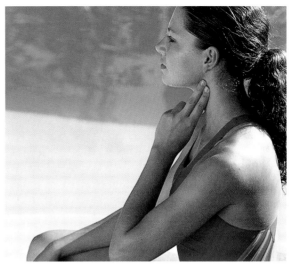

Radial pulse To check your heart rate before or during exercise, find your pulse by pressing lightly with the index and middle fingers on the radial artery on your wrist.

Carotid pulse The pulse can also be checked at the carotid artery, in the neck. In both cases, count how many pulses occur in 6 seconds, multiply by 10 and add 17.

decrease the intensity, make a fist or slice through the water. If you want to increase the frontal surface area even more, you can use webbed gloves or aquafins, both of which will increase the intensity of your workout.

Cardiovascular intensity

You will have seen people checking their heart rates while exercising. This is the easiest way to evaluate the cardiovascular intensity of the activity. There is a linear relationship between the heart rate and oxygen consumption or energy expenditure; in other words, the more energy required to perform an exercise, the faster you breathe and the faster the heart beats. In order to obtain a training effect, ACSM guidelines recommend that intensity be maintained during cardiovascular or aerobic exercise at between 55–90 percent of your maximum heart rate (220 minus your age).

In aquafitness we check the heart rate for 6 seconds instead of a full minute. When you stop exercising to check the heart rate, it decreases. On land, the heart rate of a trained individual will start to return to the pre-exercise rate within about 10 seconds of stopping

the activity. In the water, it goes down even faster, so if you check the heart rate for a full minute you won't know what the heart rate was during peak activity. In the water, the heart rate is slightly lower (by approximately 13 percent or 17 beats per minute) than the heart rate on land at an equal energy consumption. This means that you can train as hard in the water as you can on land, but your heart will not be working so hard. So when you check your heart rate, add on 17 beats per minute to your aquatic heart rate for an accurate estimate of your intensity level.

Perceived exertion

If you have a reasonable level of kinesthetic awareness — that is, the capacity to recognize and use the messages that your body sends you — you can also gauge the intensity of your workout by a subjective method known as perceived exertion. While sometimes we can over- or underestimate our capacities, usually we know pretty well what we are capable of doing. The aim is to exercise at an intensity level that will keep you breathing heavily but without suffering discomfort.

PREPARING TO WORK OUT

Over the last few pages, we've been learning about the theoretical side of aquafitness. Now it's time to put theory into practice and have some fun. But before taking the plunge, there are some practical considerations to bear in mind, to ensure that we don't overlook anything that will interrupt or ruin our workout. One of the most important of these is what to wear, and that is what we start with here, before turning to the question of posture.

CLOTHING FOR AQUAFITNESS

A swimsuit is the obvious choice when a trip to the pool is planned. But what kind of suit is best for an aquafitness workout? If you need good support, look for one with a built-in bra. Otherwise, comfort and freedom of movement are the most important factors for both men and women. For those who feel the cold, there is a variety of neoprene clothing that will help maintain body temperature in cooler water. If you intend to work out regularly, you should have at least two suits to alternate. Special fabrics have been created that are chlorine-resistant and maintain their color and elasticity despite frequent use. These may be more expensive initially but are usually worth the investment. Some people like to wear a T-shirt in the water. While this may offer some protection against sunburn, it is not a substitute for wearing a water-resistant sunblock with adequate protection for your skin type.

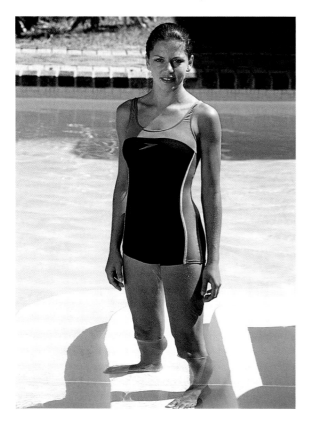

Swimsuit Freedom of movement and comfort are the main considerations, so look for a suit that does not ride up or slip off the shoulders during energetic moves.

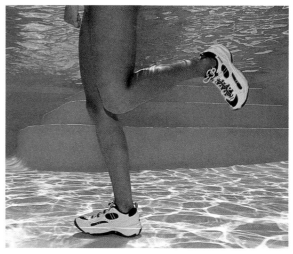

Footwear Appropriate shoes are essential in pools with a slippery or uneven surface. As well as improving stability and preventing slipping, they will protect the feet.

There are special shoes for aquafitness: some are for use exclusively in the water, while others can be used both in and out of the pool. These shoes provide traction under water and offer protection from rough pool bottoms or uneven tiles. Most aquatic shoes allow the use of arch supports during your workout, if required.

POSTURE & NEUTRAL POSITION

Your posture in water should be exactly the same as for exercise on land. When neutral position is specified, the feet should be hip-width apart, the knees extended but not locked, the pelvis in neutral alignment, abdominals contracted, chest lifted, shoulders back, and head in alignment with the back. The spine should be in neutral alignment, maintaining its four physiological curves.

There are five reference points that must be aligned vertically to ensure proper posture: these are the mastoid process (the bone behind the earlobe), the acromion process (the bony protrusion at the end of the scapula on the shoulder), the greater trocanter (the protrusion of the femur at the hip joint), the lateral collateral knee ligament (outside of the knee), and the lateral malleolus (outside of the ankle).

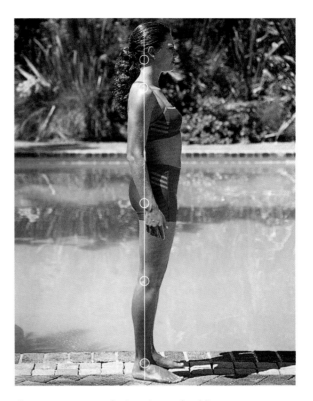

Correct posture An imaginary plumbline passes through the five reference points, which must be vertically aligned in order to ensure correct posture.

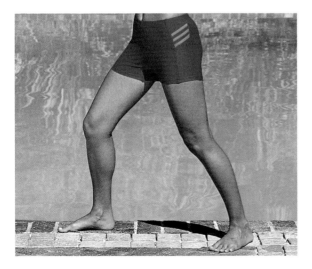

Lunge stabilizing position The legs must be at least hip-width apart, knees are slightly bent, and the feet are slightly turned out in alignment with the knees and hips.

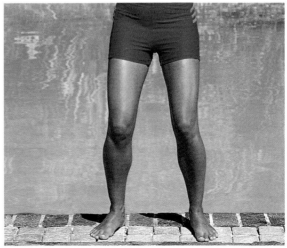

Parallel leg stabilizing position Again, the legs are hip-width apart. The feet are slightly turned out, but they are still aligned with the knees and hips.

POOL ENVIRONMENT

Before getting in the pool, familiarize yourself with the surrounding area, checking for any slippery areas where accidents could occur, as well as for steps or ladders, and indications of pool depth.

Water temperature and humidity

The ideal water temperature for aquatic fitness ranges from 82–86°F (28–30°C). Any colder, and your workout will be limited to higher intensity, aerobic, or interval-training classes. Over 86°F (30°C), it will be restricted to lower intensity, aerobic, static muscle conditioning and stretching, or Ai-Chi-type exercises. You should feel the increase in body temperature as you exercise, without becoming uncomfortably hot.

Like water temperature, humidity may not be within your control. However, be sure to keep a bottle of water at the poolside. You may not realize that you are perspiring as you work out in water, but you will, and you must replace lost fluids to prevent dehydration.

Outdoor pools

In outdoor heated pools, you may have control of the water temperature but not much else. Keep a bathrobe handy for when you get out of the water.

Pool depth, floor, and slope

Some pools range from very shallow (3 ft/90 cm and under) to deep (over 6 ft/180 cm), giving a wide choice of workout formats. In any event, you should be exercising in water that is between waist- and chest-deep, in order to protect the low back.

The pool floor may be made of various types of material, including cement, tiles, plastic, and fiberglass. Each of these has its own benefits and hazards, but the main problems for the exerciser are that the surface is either too rough or too slippery. The best way to deal with these problems is to wear aquafitness shoes, which can provide traction on a smooth floor, or protect the feet from injury on a rough surface.

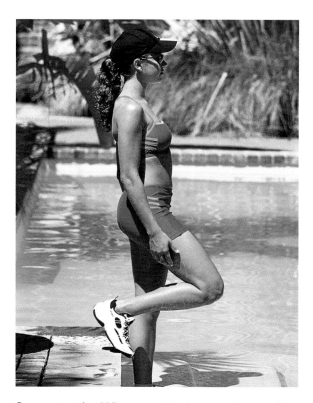

Sun protection When exercising in an outdoor pool, sunglasses are a must, as is a hat to protect the head and hair. Always apply a high-factor, water-resistant sunblock.

Another way to avoid problems with the pool floor is to work out in deep water. In this case you will need some kind of flotation device, such as a flotation belt. Another popular aid is the woggle — also known as a noodle or buoyant tube — whatever you want to call it. Whichever flotation equipment you choose, a deep-water workout is a wonderful way of exercising the whole body in a weightless environment.

For those of you fortunate enough to have a pool with varying depths, before you go in the water take note of where the slope from shallow to deep begins and how steep the slope is. Some are gradual, giving you plenty of water depths to choose from for your workout. Other pools may be shallow before suddenly plunging to deep water. It is best to be aware of this in advance, to avoid any unpleasant surprises.

USING MUSIC

Music is a great motivator for exercise, and I always urge people to work out to music if possible. Choose music with a strong beat that gives you a tempo at which to work. In class, it is the instructor's role to encourage students to exercise actively, with force and enthusiasm. When you're on your own, music can fulfill a similar motivational function.

When you chose your music, make sure that there are no interruptions between one song and the next. Your exercise workouts should be rhythmic and continuous. The speed of the song is measured in beats per minute (bpm). For aquatic fitness you can use anything in the range of 125–150 bpm, but of course the speed of the music will depend upon the depth of the water. The deeper the water, the slower the music must be because it will be more difficult to perform the movements. Also, the bigger the movements, the slower the music will have to be to give you the time to cover the full range of motion for that movement. I find that using music in the mid-tempo range works fine for all levels of fitness and all depths of water.

Choose music that you enjoy — music that moves you — and then start performing those moves that are most familiar to you. You will probably find that these have their roots in the basic steps that are described in a later chapter (*see pp34–49*). There you can find out which muscle groups you are training, and how to add other moves to create a balanced workout.

All music has a beat and it is the beat that sets the pace of the workout. Music is usually counted in four beats to a measure, but most fitness instructors count eight beats, because eight movements are usually performed in one measure of music. In fact, the basic unit of the movement combination is called an "eight-count." This works fine on land, but in water, resistance can make this speed of movement more difficult.

As you follow the programs at the end of the book, or put together your own workouts, listen to music either on a battery-operated tape deck or CD player near the pool or, if you are in a public pool, you can use a waterproof personal cassette or CD player.

Choosing a tempo

Most exercises are best performed at water and half-water tempo (*see box*). Play around with the moves and the music so that you get used to working on the beat. Your moves should be big and controlled, but initially your main problem will be keeping your feet on the ground while staying on the beat. Start by moving in a smaller range of motion and gradually increase the range of motion and intensity as you become stronger and more accustomed to working in the water.

Some of the workouts in this book are based choreographically on the variation of tempos between water, half-water with a bounce, half-water with a hold, and some land tempo. It is worth becoming familiar with different tempos and learning how to use them to add variety and enjoyment to your workout.

EXERCISING TO A TEMPO

Land tempo
In an eight-count of music, you can perform four complete jogs, made up of eight different movements.

1	2	3	4	5	6	7	8
Jog R	Jog L	Jog R	Jog L	Jog R	Jog L	Jog R	Jog L

Water tempo
In an eight-count of music, you perform two complete jogs, made up of four different movements.

1–2	3–4	5–6	7–8
Jog R	Jog L	Jog R	Jog L

Half-water tempo with a bounce
Here you perform one complete jog, uniting the feet between each of the two movements.

1–2	3–4	5–6	7–8
Jog R	Unite feet	Jog L	Unite feet

Half-water tempo with a hold
Here you perform one complete jog, holding the position between each of the two movements

1–2	3–4	5–6	7–8
Jog R	Hold	Jog L	Hold

BUOYANCY AND FLOTATION EQUIPMENT

On land, weights are used to increase the workload on the muscles. In water, however, we are working in a weightless environment and using weights would be counterproductive. Instead, we use the water and its characteristics to find different ways of challenging ourselves in order to become stronger and fitter.

Buoyancy equipment

As is clear from our discussion of buoyancy (*see p11*), buoyancy equipment is anything that floats in water. It is used vertically against the force of buoyancy, in exactly the opposite way that weights are used on land. On land, when you lift a weight against the force of gravity, you are working with your biceps muscle. In the water, working against the force of buoyancy, you will be pushing the equipment downward, working the triceps muscle group. This is an interesting concept: in the water, we work all the muscle groups that are difficult to work on land because there, they are assisted by gravity. Buoyancy equipment is available with different levels of resistance. The woggle, or noodle, for example, offers a light resistance and is suitable for

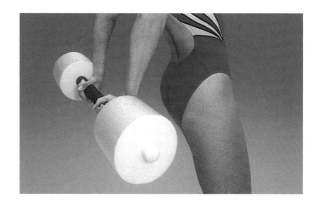

The swimbar gives added resistance to any downward movement, due to its density. Buoyant equipment works vertically, in opposition to the force of gravity.

initial resistance training. As you get stronger, you may want to invest in a set of handbars, which are available in various densities, or resistances; then you may want to move on to the swimbar, the closed chain disk, and finally, my favorite — the kickroller. Both of the last two aids originated in physical therapy, but have adapted well to the needs of the aquafitness community.

When using buoyancy equipment, you must keep your feet on the ground at all times. Your strength and capabilities will determine the type and density of

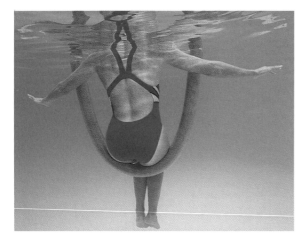

The buoyant noodle can be used as a flotation device. Sitting on it, as shown here, will keep the exerciser afloat. Arms are out to the sides to stabilize.

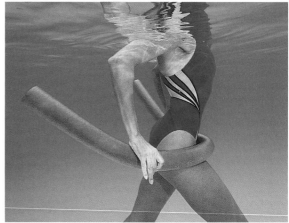

When it is being pushed back and forth in front of the body, as well as being held down, the buoyant noodle functions as drag as well as buoyant equipment.

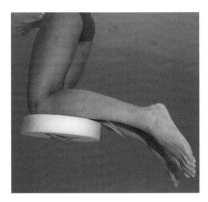

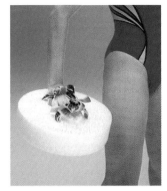

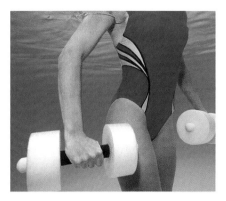

The closed chain disk, on which the exerciser is kneeling, is being used here as a flotation aid while training balance and core stability.

Pushing the closed chain disk down takes advantage of the larger frontal surface area to increase muscular intensity.

Just holding the handbars under the water, without moving them, gives an isometric workout for the lats, pecs, and triceps muscles.

equipment that you use. Your abdominals and back muscles must work very hard to stabilize your trunk so that the equipment isn't pushing you around. Remember that you are in charge – you must use the equipment and not let it use you! If you get tired, quit! There is no sense in getting injured. You can alternate working with and without equipment as in an aerobic circuit training program (*see p150*), or you can use a lighter density piece of equipment, or you can try working in shallower water (always keeping the low back protected by working in at least waist-deep water.)

When using buoyant equipment, keep the wrist in neutral alignment – that is, in a straight line from hand to the forearm. Never bend it down or back, as this can cause stress to the wrist joint, with resultant pain.

When pushing equipment down against the force of gravity, maintain the spine in neutral alignment and do not hunch up the shoulders in order to force down the arms. Never sacrifice alignment to perform an exercise.

Flotation equipment

Flotation equipment is usually the same as buoyancy equipment – it is just used differently. While the latter is employed against the vertical force of buoyancy, we use flotation equipment to keep us afloat in the water.

In this case, the equipment is used not so much to overload your body as to support you in a suspended state so that you can do other things. The one piece of flotation equipment used exclusively to keep you afloat is the flotation belt. There are several on the market, but you must find one that is most comfortable for your body shape. You will find information on the manufacturers and suppliers of the equipment used in this book on p157.

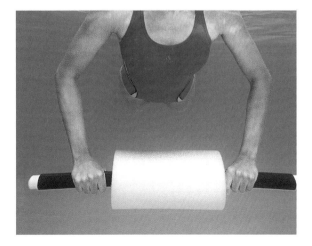

Push-ups in deep water not only work your chest and arms; you will be using your abdominals and glutes to stay horizontal and training your balance at the same time.

DRAG EQUIPMENT

This equipment increases the surface area of the body part moving in the water, thus increasing the resistance. It can be used in every direction In the water, unlike buoyancy equipment, which works only vertically. Drag equipment is effective only when the body part with the equipment is moving through the water, again unlike buoyancy equipment, which continuously tries to reach the surface whether you are moving or not.

Drag doesn't depend only on the surface area, however; it also depends on the shape of the object, the speed of the movement, the density of the water, its turbulence, and the projected surface area, amongst other factors. There are many ways of using drag equipment to modify the intensity of the exercise, but one particular benefit is that it ensures muscle balance by working both sides of the muscle pair equally. For example, in bending the elbow you work the biceps muscle; on the return movement, straightening the arm, you work the triceps muscle.

Since drag resistance is felt in every direction in which there is movement, some pieces of buoyant equipment can also be used for drag, giving you a double workout: firstly, in holding the equipment under the water against buoyancy, and secondly, by pushing it through the water against the water's resistance.

It is important to remember that the elbows and knees and other joints involved in the movement should be neither locked nor hyperextended, but always remain soft and slightly flexed. The drag forces should be experienced by the muscles — not by the joints, which should always be protected.

Webbed gloves

Webbed gloves are the most popular kind of drag equipment on the market. The webbing between the fingers turn your hands into "paddles" with an increased frontal surface area. Webbed gloves come in various materials, including latex, Lycra, and neoprene. Your choice of gloves can make a difference to your workout,

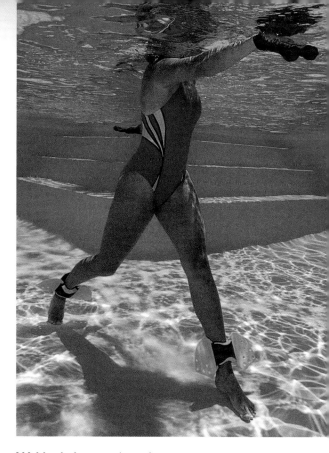

Webbed gloves and aquafins are typical examples of drag equipment. By increasing the frontal surface area, they increase the intensity of the movement.

so try on different types before you buy and choose a pair that feels right for you. My preference is for Lycra, which is soft and malleable — you will hardly notice that you're wearing Lycra gloves, but you will definitely feel the difference when you move your hands in the water. Many of my clients prefer neoprene, which gives a stronger resistance and lasts longer.

Aquafins

This is another very effective piece of drag equipment, which can be worn on either the wrists or the ankles. Aquafins look like wings and notably increase drag resistance in opposition to the direction of the movement of the limbs. Depending on which exercise is being performed, they can be adjusted to point from front to back or from side to side in order to increase the relevant frontal surface area.

Elastic bands

Elastic bands and tubing serve a dual purpose in the water. The first and primary purpose is to increase the intensity of movements. Once you are familiar with your water workout, you will know how much force you need to apply in order to move an arm or leg. Using elastic bands or tubing in the water will allow you to perform many of the same exercises with more intensity by adding the resistance of the band or tubing to the water's resistance.

The second purpose of using elastic bands and tubing is to work certain muscle groups in ways they cannot otherwise be exercised in water. For examples of these, see the photographs below.

When using elastic bands or tubes, one end is held or fixed, while at the other end, the arm or leg moves to stretch out the equipment, thereby increasing the intensity or difficulty of the move. As with drag equipment, the movement can be in any direction, but you will have to control the return part of the muscle contraction. For example, let's say that you are holding one end of the band in one hand in an isometric contraction and with the other arm you are performing a biceps curl. As the band stretches while performing the curl, the intensity increases; once you begin the return to the initial position, you will have to control the band to prevent it from pulling your other arm back down. This controlled resistance to the band's return involves an eccentric contraction (*see p14*), which is a component of the muscle contraction that cannot be obtained in water without the use of equipment. An eccentric contraction is also achieved when using buoyancy equipment, in controlling the return of such equipment to the surface of the water.

Complete your workout

Elastic tubing and bands can also be used on land, where you can perform exercises for the triceps, the latissimus dorsi, and the trapezius muscle groups that cannot be performed in water. This enables you to keep your workout complete, if you want to include these particular exercises in your aquafitness program.

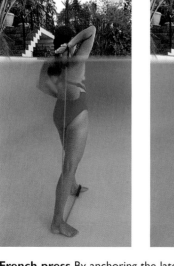 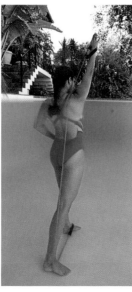 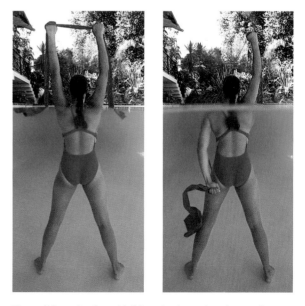

French press By anchoring the latex tubing under the foot, you can still extend the arm over the head and use the triceps muscle in a French press.

Exercising the lats Holding the latex band over the head and then pulling one end down behind the back exercises the lats in a full range of motion.

THE WORKOUT STRUCTURE

The warmup is the most important part of the workout. Performed in the water, and usually lasting from 8–10 minutes, it consists of a balanced combination of rhythmic, limbering movements, similar to those of the workout, interspersed with stretches for the major muscle groups. During the warmup, move continuously to keep the heart rate and body temperature elevated.

A typical warmup might include: 16 front kneelifts with complementary arms; 16 jumping jacks with bilateral shoulder rotation; 16 jogs with complementary arms; a low back stretch; 16 hopscotches with shoulder pullbacks and front crossovers; arms above the head for a lat stretch on the right side, then on the left. Continue with jog to kick, alternating legs 16 times; right leg back in a quad and iliopsoas stretch; jog 8 times, then left leg back for a quad and iliopsoas stretch. Kick the legs forward into front quad kicks 16 times; right leg up in front to stretch out the back of the leg; repeat the front quad kicks 16 times, then repeat the hamstring and calf stretch on the left leg. (*See The Basic Moves, pp34–49.*) A warmup will initiate any and every exercise program. Once the warmup is complete, start on the main part of your workout.

Workout

There are several types of workout formats to choose from. In aquafitness, these may be performed in shallow or deep water, thus doubling the choice available.

The Aerobic Bell Curve is basically a workout format for cardiovascular or aerobic exercise. After the initial warmup, the intensity gradually increases until you reach a level that can be maintained for at least 20 minutes. After this, you gradually decrease the intensity until you have returned to your pre-exercise heart rate.

A Muscle Conditioning workout includes exercises in sets and repetitions. Such a format would probably use some kind of equipment in order to overload the muscles being trained. The number of sets and repetitions is chosen on the basis of the needs of the exerciser as well as on his or her capabilities.

In a **Circuit Training** format, the exerciser executes a number of repetitions of an exercise, then immediately goes on to another exercise for another body part. This format maintains the cardiovascular activity so that some aerobic benefits can be obtained by this method.

Aerobic Circuit Training combines an aerobic workout with a circuit workout. It is divided into cycles or time periods, which will vary according to the individual goals and objectives of the exerciser. During each cycle, an aerobic interval at mid- to high-intensity level is alternated with an active recovery interval of 1.5 minutes of muscle-conditioning exercises.

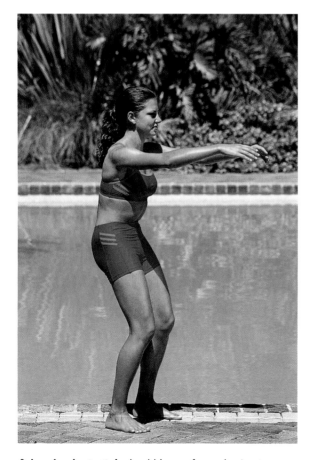

A low back stretch should be performed prior to any twisting or lateral bending. Keeping the shoulders back and down, contract the abdominals, and do a pelvic tilt.

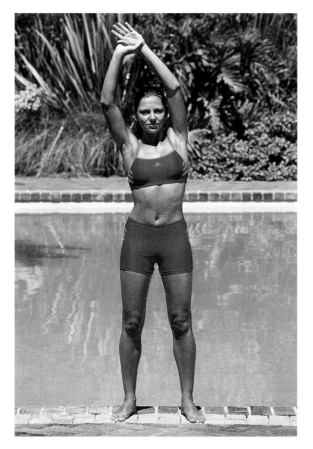

Latissimus dorsi stretch To elongate your left lat, pull your left hand above your right shoulder with the right hand, and vice versa. The shoulders are back and down.

Interval Training is a specifically cardiovascular workout format. It involves exercising at very high intensity rates, then performing active recovery at lower intensity rates. The activity may be the same throughout, but the intensity rate is not. The purpose of this kind of exercise is to increase your anaerobic threshold — that is, the intensity level over which lactic acid accumulates in the muscles and liver. While interval training is directly linked to high intensity exercise by professional athletes, it can also be used for beginners or novice exercisers, who will alternate periods of more intense exercise with less intense recovery exercises, such as "cycling" faster and slower in deep water.

Stretching and Relaxation workouts are geared to flexibility and joint mobility and, for this reason, water temperatures must be warmer. Suitable formats include Watsu® (*see pp118–121*) or Ai Chi (*see pp110–117*), or exercises for special populations (*see p155*) After the warmup, movements continue to be rhythmic and expansive in order to maintain the body temperature, which is assisted here by warmer water temperatures.

Cooldown

At the end of each workout, we need time to return to our pre-exercise state. We continue the movements executed during the workout, but now they become less intense. Again we include static and dynamic stretching of the major muscles used during the workout to increase overall flexibility and joint mobility.

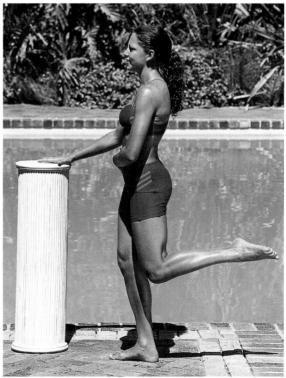

To stretch the quads and iliopsoas, bend the knee and pull the leg back, thrusting the hip forward. Keep the abdominals contracted and the supporting knee soft.

CONTRAINDICATIONS TO AQUAFITNESS

While there aren't many contraindications to aquafitness, there are a number of conditions where caution is advisable. Always seek medical advice before embarking on an aquafitness or any exercise program. In each of the exercise combinations in the book, we include advice on movements that should be avoided or limited to avoid strain on vulnerable areas.

MEDICAL CONDITIONS

It is always a good idea to check with your physician before you begin an exercise program. This is particularly relevant if you have a history of cardiovascular problems, pulmonary disease, musculoskeletal disorders, or hypertension. If you suffer from any of these conditions, please seek medical advice before embarking on an aquafitness program. Other possible contraindications include open skin wounds, allergy to chlorine, skin infections or contagious conditions, and fever. The needs of special populations, such as seniors and pregnant women, are discussed on p155.

While it is very unlikely that anyone will drown while doing aquafitness, there are people who are afraid of being in deep water, where they cannot touch the bottom. In this case, I suggest they limit themselves to exercising in waist- to rib-depth water (in order to protect the low back) and stay near the edge of the pool. Over time, and with familiarity, most people gain confidence and lose their fear of the water.

Low blood pressure is not necessary a contraindication to aquafitness, but overdoing exercise in the water may accentuate the condition. Never work on a completely empty stomach and, if you feel dizzy or nauseous, stop. Be particularly careful if the air and/or water temperature are warmer than usual and you are working out with particular intensity.

It is important that an exerciser with epilepsy is accompanied by someone who knows about their condition and can intervene in the event of a seizure.

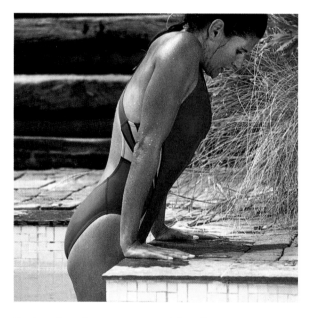

Pectoral push-ups may cause injury if you are not strong enough to maintain perfect alignment while pulling yourself up. These are best performed on land.

CONTRAINDICATED EXERCISES

These are exercises that may cause some damage to the body when repeated. Often, they are familiar exercises that "everybody does." In the past, we did not have the research or the means to study the stress under which we place our muscles, joints, tendons, and ligaments when exercising. Now that science can confirm the risk involved, let's learn which exercises are best avoided or see how to modify them so that you can get the benefits without the risk of injury.

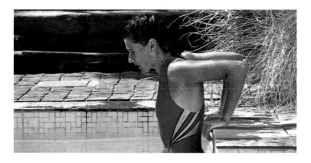

Triceps dips Struggling to pull the body out of the water, with shoulders hunched and elbows blocked or even hyperextended, is best avoided.

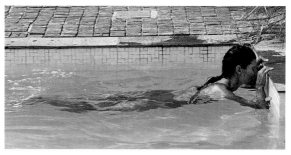

Prone flutter kicks cause the exerciser to hyperextend both the low back and the neck, increasing the risk of injury to both of those areas. Don't do them!

Muscle conditioning

We have illustrated here some of the exercises that you will have seen people doing in the pool. All of these should be avoided because they are more likely to cause strain and injury than to tone the muscles.

Aerobics

There are a number of movements that should be avoided because of the risk injury or strain:

Very high impact continuous movement, where the body is propelled out of the water during rebound. This is especially true in shallower water. People usually work out in water to avoid the stress that comes from the force of gravity and high impact forces. High intensity can be achieved without high impact.

Very fast movements or even movements at land tempo. Exercise in water requires slower movements in order to overcome the water's resistance and maintain proper alignment. To perform the exercises safely at land tempo, you will have to reduce the range of motion, which reduces the effectiveness of the workout.

Using the arms continuously above the head will stimulate the "pressor response." This occurs when, in order to push the blood against gravity to the arms and hands, the heart must beat harder and faster. Continuously moving the arms overhead can also cause injury to the shoulder joint.

Moving the arms in and out of the water during exercise can cause injury to the shoulder joint, because of the phenomenon of surface tension.

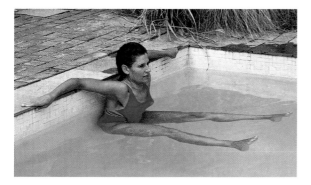

Wall-hanging exercises put your shoulder joint under extreme stress, as well as putting strain on the wrists and elbows. Again, best avoided.

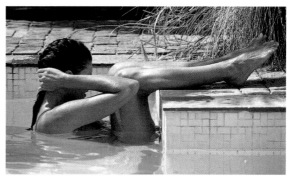

Wall-hanging sit-ups do not exercise the abdominals. If you want to do sit-ups, do them on land – or check out the abdominal exercises that can be done in water.

THE BASIC MOVES

In this chapter, you will learn the basic steps and movements that are used in aquafitness, including those that you'll encounter in later sections of the book. Here I explain in detail what to do with your arms and legs in order to exercise your body in a safe and effective way, in both shallow and deep water. Just for fun, try doing the exercises with the music at water tempo and half-water tempo (*see p25*).

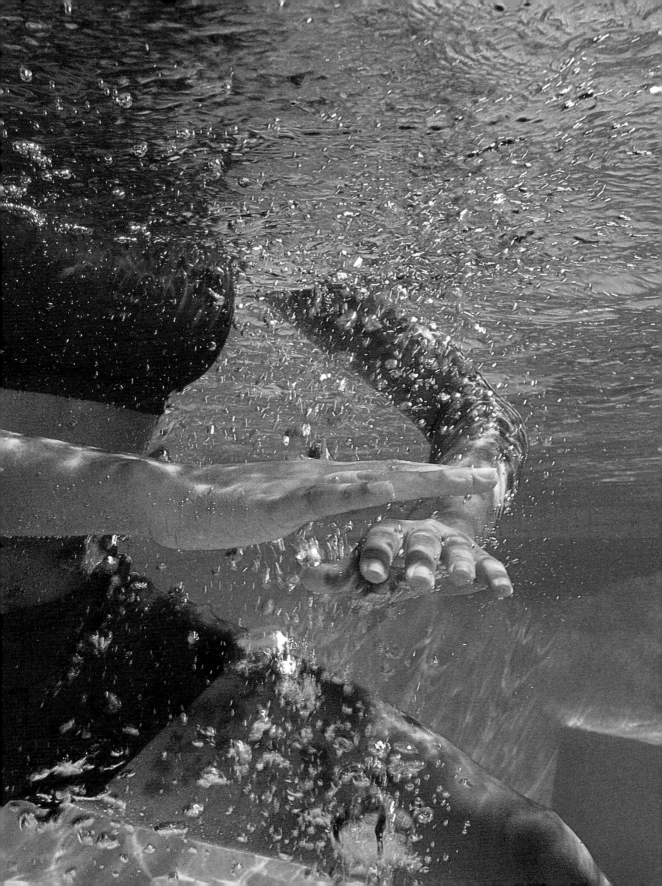

ARM POSITIONS

The arms can be used to complement your movements, easing the intensity of the exercise or increasing it. You can hold your arms out to the sides to help stabilize your body or use them in the five basic movements described on this and the following pages to exercise parts of the trunk and upper body. Remember to keep your arms under the water at all times – it's the only way to tone the arm, shoulder, chest, and back muscles.

COMPLEMENTARY MOVEMENTS

In aquafitness, the arms play an important role in the execution of the exercises. You will come across the term "complementary arm movements;" by this we mean moves that assist leg movements. For example, in a jog, when you lift your right foot back, the right hand comes forward and the left hand goes back. If you extend your left foot forward, your right hand will naturally come forward. This is called opposition. It is natural. When complementary arms are indicated, do what comes naturally – what seems easy and requires no thought. Your attention will be on the lower body but, whenever you move your arms, you will be toning the upper body muscles at the same time.

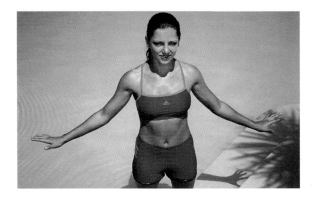

Stabilizing arm position It is easiest to maintain your balance in the water when the arms are held out to the sides, with the hands gently sculling the water. Keep the shoulder blades back and down when you raise the arms.

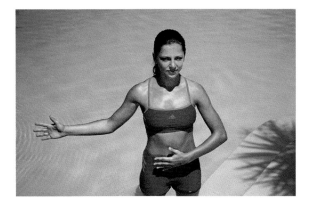

Performing a different move with each arm is known as unilateral, or asymmetrical, movement. In the example above, the model has turned her right arm out to the side, while her left arm turns inward. This will be followed by turning the left arm out and the right arm in.

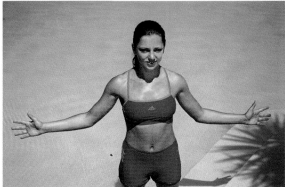

Performing the same move with each arm is known as bilateral, or symmetrical, movement. In the example above, the model has turned both of her arms out to the sides. This will be followed by turning both arms inward, in another bilateral movement.

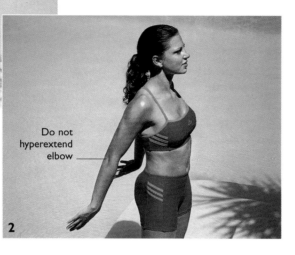

Palms
toward
body

Do not
hyperextend
elbow

I

2

BENDING & EXTENDING THE ELBOWS

This movement works the biceps and triceps muscles (*see pp92–93*) by alternately bending and extending the elbows. Starting with the arms by the sides, bend the elbows and bring the open hands up toward the shoulders. Palms face toward the body **I**.

Straighten the elbows, extending the arms behind you, with the palms facing back **2**. Do not hyperextend the elbows.

You may vary the exercise by bending the right elbow as the left arm straightens, and vice versa. Keep the hands under the water and work in a full range of motion.

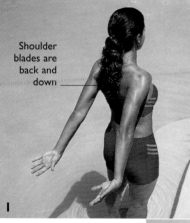

Shoulder
blades are
back and
down

I

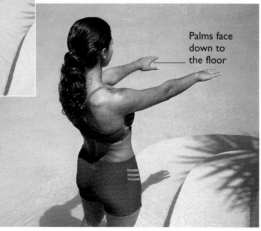

Palms face
down to
the floor

2

SHOULDER FRONT RAISES & PRESSBACKS

Here, the movement occurs at the shoulder joint as the arms move forward and back, working the anterior and posterior delts, pecs, and lats (*see pp94–97*). Again, we show the arms working bilaterally, but the move can also be performed with one arm to the front and the other to the back, as you do when cross-country skiing.

Starting in neutral position, with the hands by the sides, extend both arms to the back. Hands are open with the palms facing back **I**.

With the palms facing down, swing the arms forward until they are parallel to the floor **2**. Shoulder blades are back and down as you swing the arms back and forth.

▶

Arms out to the
side at shoulder
level

Shoulder
blades back
and down

I

SHOULDER LATERAL RAISES & PULLDOWNS

In the previous exercises, we moved the arms back and forth. Now we take them out to the sides, working the medial deltoids and latissimus dorsi muscles (see pp14–15). Starting in neutral position, with the arms down by the sides, raise both arms out to the sides at shoulder height **I**.

Return to neutral position with your arms down by your sides **2**.

You can vary the hand position for this exercise. For example, they may be palm down when the arms are extended, as shown here, or palm up, or alternately palm up and palm down. Keep the hands and arms under the water in all positions.

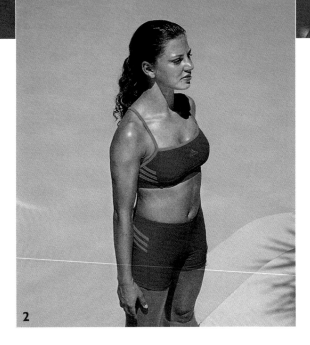

2

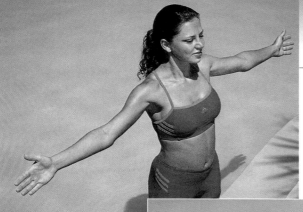

1

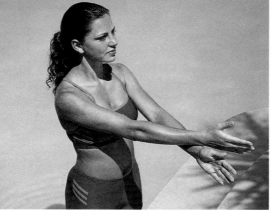

2

SHOULDER PULLBACKS & FRONT CROSSOVERS

Start with the arms out to the sides at shoulder height (under the water, of course). The hands are open, with the palms facing forward **1**.

Keeping your arms at the same height, bring them forward until they cross at the wrists **2**.

This movement, which works the pectoralis major and trapezius muscles (*see pp14–15*), will force you to contract your abdominal and back muscles to stabilize the trunk and stop you from being pushed back and forth in the water as you move your arms.

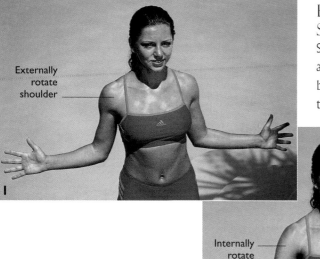

Externally rotate shoulder

1

Internally rotate shoulder

2

EXTERNAL/INTERNAL SHOULDER ROTATION

Start in neutral position, with your back straight, arms by your sides, and your shoulder blades back and down. Bend the elbows and turn out the arms, keeping the elbows close to the body. The hands are open, with palms facing forward **1**.

Turn the arms inward until the hands overlap in front of the body **2**. You will feel the contraction between the shoulder blades. Avoid hunching your back and raising your shoulders as you move your arms forward.

KNEELIFT AND KICK

Both kneelifts and kicks involve similar hip movements – the difference is in the movement of the knee. A kneelift is performed with the knee bent, while in a kick, the leg is straight. Both moves involve muscle masses that are particularly important for cardiovascular and muscular fitness, and it is for this reason that they and their many variations are among the most commonly used movements in aquafitness.

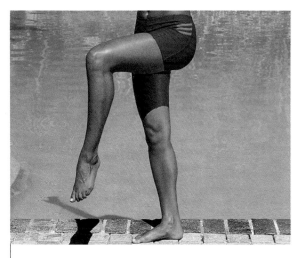

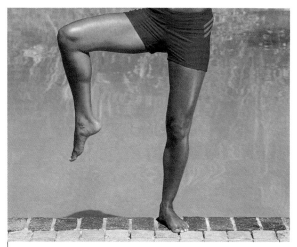

FRONT KNEELIFT
Starting from neutral position, with the feet hip-width apart, the knees soft, and the shoulders back and down, raise the left leg directly in front of the body until the thigh is parallel to the floor. The left foot points directly downward. As the left leg returns to the original position, the right leg performs the kneelift. In all the kneelift variations, try to maintain hip-knee-foot alignment.

SIDE KNEELIFT
Turn the right leg out and raise it to the side until the thigh is parallel to the floor. Repeat with the left leg. Keep the support leg slightly bent.

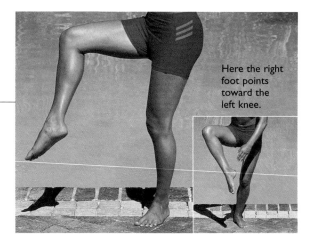

Here the right foot points toward the left knee.

OPEN KNEELIFT
In this variation, the right leg is turned out and lifted in a diagonal position that is halfway between a front and a side kneelift. The foot can either point straight down to the floor, or in toward the opposite knee (*inset*). As the right leg returns to the original position, the left leg repeats the kneelift.

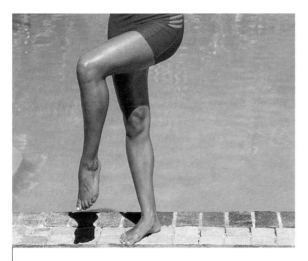

CROSSOVER KNEELIFT
In another variation of the kneelift, the flexed left leg is pulled across the midline as it is raised in front of the body. As you return the left leg to neutral position, raise the right leg in a crossover kneelift. Keep the supporting knee soft at all times.

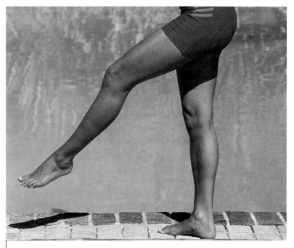

QUAD KICK
Starting with the left leg raised in a front kneelift, straighten it out into a kick and point the foot. You can repeat the kneelift and kick several times before lowering the leg, or alternate quad kicks on either side. This kick can start from any kneelift position.

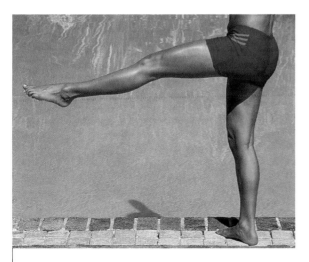

HIGH KICK
In the high kick, the entire leg is raised from the starting position. It can be performed in many directions and in different ways: directly forward, sideways, diagonally across the midline, or diagonally outward. Whichever variation you choose, repeat the movements equally with both legs.

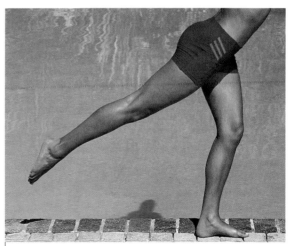

BACK KICK
This variation uses the gluteus maximus; the hip flexors are not involved. Contract the abdominals and stabilize the low back, raising the leg only as high as is comfortable, either straight toward the back or diagonally outward. Repeat equally on both sides, and avoid locking the support knee.

BOUNCE, JOG, AND HOPSCOTCH

Now we have three more basic steps, all of which may be familiar to you from land-based exercises. The hard part in all of them is keeping your feet on the ground or, in the case of deep water, keeping your feet pointed toward the pool bottom while you work. The jog and the hopscotch work the muscles on the back of the thigh (the hamstrings), while the bounce works the quads, the hamstrings, and the calf muscles.

BOUNCE

Start in neutral position, with the feet hip-width apart and the knees soft 1.

Flexing the hips and knees, and using your arms to help push you upward, lift both feet off the pool floor 2. Straighten the legs and use the arms to help you return to the starting position. The size of the bounce can vary from a heel lift to a tuck jump, as here, and can be done with legs together or apart.

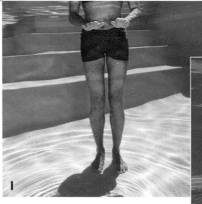
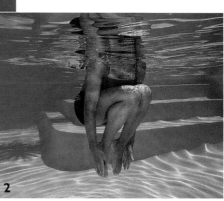

JOG

Starting in neutral position, bend the right knee and lift the leg up behind the body. The knee remains directly under the hip and in alignment with the shoulder. The right arm pushes forward and the left goes back 1.

As the leg straightens to return to the starting position, bring the left leg up behind the body and push the left arm forward 2. Keep the abdominals contracted as you jog to protect the low back, and be careful not to raise the foot so high behind you that it causes you to arch your back.

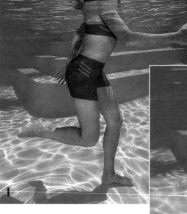
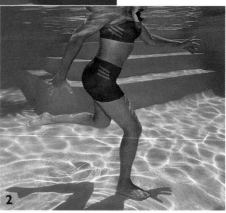

HOPSCOTCH

Start from neutral position, with feet hip-width apart. Bend the right knee and turn the leg out at the hip so the knee points outward and the foot comes up behind the supporting leg **1**.

Return to the starting position, with the feet apart and the knees soft. Arms are out to the sides in a stabilizing position **2**.

Repeat the movement on the other side, bending the left knee and turning out the left leg **3**.

To increase the intensity, hop directly from one leg to the other, missing out the neutral position in between (water tempo). Otherwise, return to the neutral position between hops (half-water tempo, see p25).

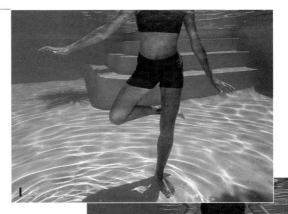

1

2

3

SIDE STEP, JUMPING JACKS, AND HIP-HOP JACKS

After the front-to-back exercises on the previous spread, we turn to three moves that work the abductor and adductor muscle groups (*see pp102–103*). These are the muscles that move the legs out to the sides and in again, so these exercise are a great way to tone your thighs. The side step is the base from which subsequent movements stem.

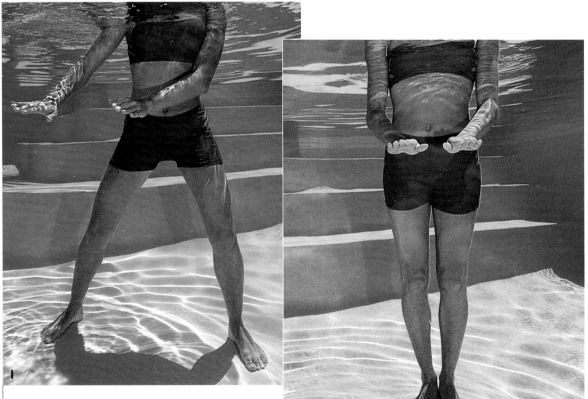

SIDE STEP

Start from neutral position, with the feet together. Move the right leg out to the side **1**.

Bring the left leg in to meet the right, returning to the starting position **2**. This exercise can be done in both directions. The side step can be performed as a low-impact exercise by keeping one foot in contact with the pool floor at all times. Increase intensity to high impact by hopping as you open the feet. Contract your abdominals and use your arms to help push you in the direction of movement.

JUMPING JACKS

Start in neutral position, with the legs together **1**.

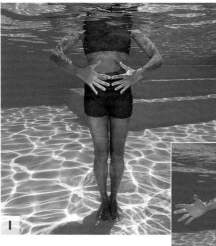

Hop and open the legs to the sides **2**. Return to the starting position with another hop. The arms open to the sides as the legs open, and close to the front as the legs come together. Keep the hands under water.

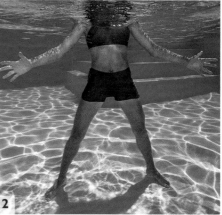

Crossover Jack Increase the range of the movement by crossing the legs over on the return, instead of landing with the feet together.

Aquatic Air Jack In this variation, the legs should reach the fully open position while afloat, and come together before landing in neutral position — either with the feet together or in the crossover position.

HIP-HOP JACK

Starting from neutral position, with the legs together, hop and open the legs to the sides **1**.

With another hop, pull the legs in and tuck them up under the body **2**.

Now straighten the legs and take them out to the sides again to land. While you are in the tucked position the water will support you, allowing you to pull up your legs and contract your abdominals, thus relaxing the low back. Your arms and hands push out and pull in to assist the leg movements.

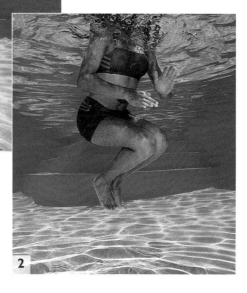

This is a great exercise, working the inner thighs during the tuck jump and exercising the glutes as you straighten and lower your legs.

STRIDE, LUNGE, PENDULUM, AND TIC-TOC

Another four movements that give a great workout, as well as being fun to do. The first two are back and forth movements, toning and conditioning the gluteal muscles. The pendulum and tic-toc work the inner and outer thighs with their side-to-side movements. Keep the abdominal muscles tight to protect the low back while you exercise.

STRIDE

Start from neutral position, with the feet under the hips. Keeping the knees slightly bent, hop and stride the right leg forward and the left leg back **1**.

Hopping again, change sides, bringing the left leg forward and the right leg back **2**. The arms are complementary, working in opposition to the legs. opposition to the legs.

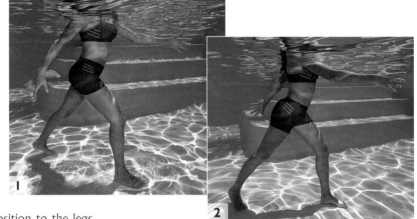

LUNGE

Start from neutral position, with the feet under the hips. Keeping the support leg slightly bent, hop and stretch the right leg to the rear. The ball of the foot is on the floor but the heel is off the ground **1**.

Hop back to neutral position **2**.

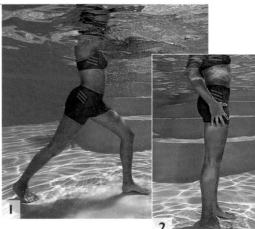

Repeat on the opposite side, extending the left leg to the rear **3**. The arms push forward as the working leg goes back, and pull in to the hips as you return to neutral. Lunges can also be performed to the front and to the side.

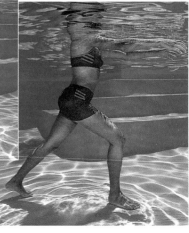

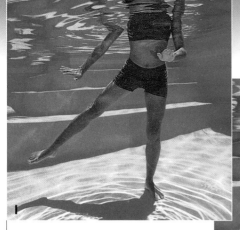

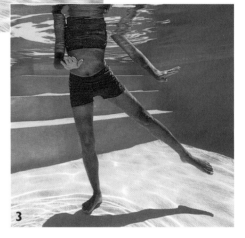

PENDULUM

Start in neutral position, with the feet under the hips. Hop and raise the right leg out to the side, with the knee facing forward. The right arm pushes out with the right leg **1**.

With another hop, return to the starting position **2**.

Repeat the movement with the left leg, hopping and raising the left leg **3**. Continue hopping and opening, then hopping and closing the legs. This is half-water tempo with a bounce (*see p25*). The pendulum can be performed at half-water tempo by holding the leg out to the side for three beats before raising the other leg; or at water tempo by opening the leg to the side in two beats as the other leg returns to center.

TIC-TOC

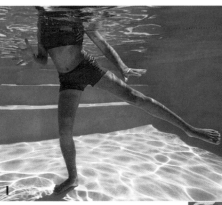

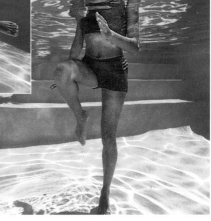

Start in neutral position, with the feet under the hips. Hop and raise the left leg to the side **1**. You will be traveling to the right.

Hopping again, bring the left leg back to the starting position. At the same time, raise the right leg in a front kneelift **2**. Hop and raise the left leg to the side, and continue alternating side leg raises and front kneelifts for 4–8 complete repetitions. (A complete repetition includes one side leg raise and one front kneelift.)

The tic-toc may be performed on both sides. The arms will help push you in the direction in which you are traveling.

TWIST, ROCKING HORSE, AND GAZELLE

Time now to let your imagination fly. We start off with an aquatic version of that old favorite, the twist, which tones the abdominal muscles. Next, it's back to the playroom for rocking horses, a fantastic move for improving cardiovascular fitness. Then it's up in the clouds, leaping like a gazelle, to increase hip mobility.

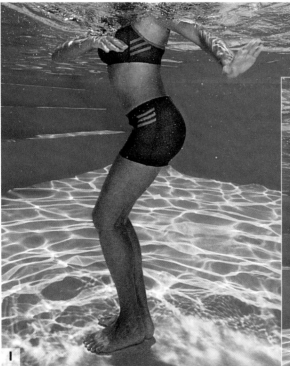

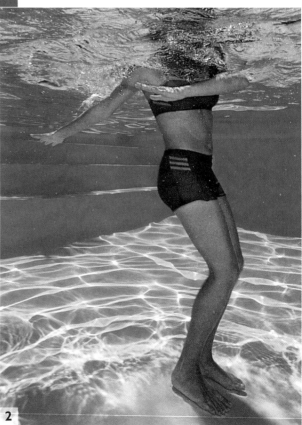

TWIST,

Stand in neutral position, with the legs together or hip-width apart and the knees soft. To protect the back, contract the abdominals and elongate the spine to maintain the correct distance between the vertebrae. Hop and twist the upper body to the left and the lower body to the right **1**. The arms move in the opposite direction of the lower body.

Hopping again, twist the upper body to the right and the lower body to the left, returning to the starting position or continuing to complete the twist in the opposite direction **2**.

ROCKING HORSE

Stand in neutral position, with the feet under the hips and the knees soft. Lean back slightly and raise the right leg in a front kneelift **1**.

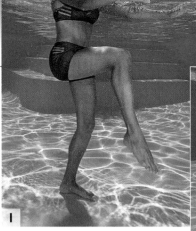

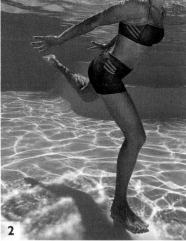

As you bring the right leg down to the floor, lean forward slightly and bend the left leg back in a jog **2**. As the left leg returns to the floor, bring the right leg back into a front kneelift and continue rocking back and forth for at least four complete repetitions. Repeat on the other side, starting with a left front kneelift. The arms can either complement or oppose the movements.

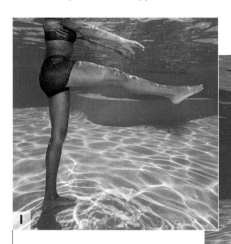

GAZELLE

Stand in neutral position, with the feet under the hips and the knees soft. Raise the right leg in a front kneelift, then extend the leg forward **1**. Both arms reach out to the front, bilaterally, or you can work with complementary arms, unilaterally (*see p36*).

As you extend the right leg, push yourself off the floor with the left leg **2**. (In deep water, you will have to push off against the water.) The outstretched arms move from front to back to help you glide through the water. The back leg can either be extended, as in a split, or bent, as in a hurdler's jump.

The left leg then comes forward into a front kneelift, ready for another leap, this time leading with the left leg **3**. As you push off, imagine that you are as light and graceful as a gazelle.

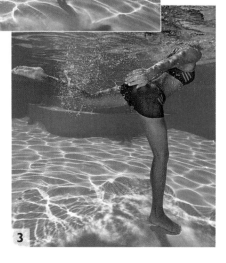

SHALLOW-WATER

COMBINATIONS

Now that you know the basic moves of aquafitness, let's put them together in combinations: this is a sequence of basic movements performed in counts of eight beats. Each combination, which is worked in rib- to shoulder-depth water, starts with a simple repetitive movement, to which we add on further steps and drop off previous repetitions. Suggested number of repetitions are given throughout, but you can vary these to suit your fitness level or time available. To increase intensity, you can wear aquafins or webbed gloves for any of these combinations (*see pp 28–29*). Don't forget to start with a warmup (*see p30*) and end with a cooldown (*see p31*).

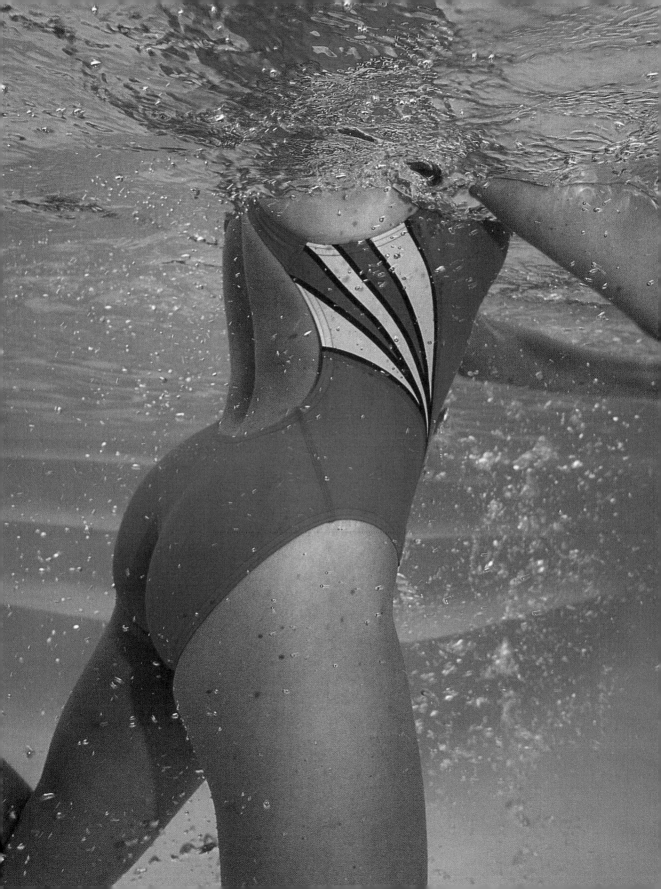

STAR 1

Using a variety of moves, including the kneelift, kick, jog, and hopscotch, the Star combinations form the core of our shallow-water exercises. We will move the legs in all directions – front, back, and sides, as well as in internal and external rotation – increasing hip mobility and toning muscles.

CAUTION: When you extend the leg back in the stride, keep the back heel off the ground and contract the abdominals to protect the low back. Never hyperextend the knees. Raise the leg only as far as is comfortable for you.

INTENSITY: Increase the intensity by using more force with the arms and the legs on the strides.

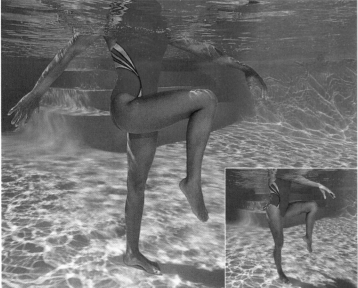

2 **FRONT KICK.** Start as in Step 1. After the third right kneelift, extend the right leg into a front kick. Repeat on the other side. Continue for at least eight repetitions. Repeat the combination on the right, then bend and extend the knee twice for a total of three kicks. Repeat, starting with a front kneelift to the left. Continue for at least four repetitions.

1 **FRONT KNEELIFT.** Starting from neutral position, with the feet hip-width apart, raise the right knee in front of the body. Repeat with the left knee, and continue alternating sides for at least eight complete repetitions. (A complete repetition includes a front kneelift with both legs.) The foot of the working leg points down to the floor, and the arms are complementary, working in opposition to the legs.

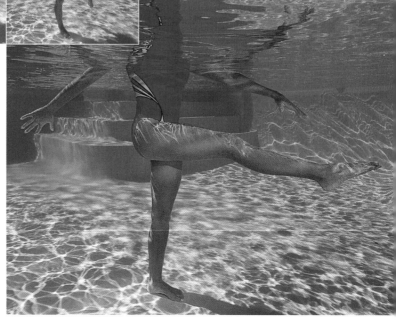

3 STRIDE. Bring the leg that has just kicked (here the right) back into a stride, pushing it down and back to the extended position. Keep the back heel off the ground. The entire supporting foot remains in contact with the floor. During the strides, the arms are complementary, pushing back and forth in opposition to the legs. Stride for four complete repetitions. (A complete repetition includes a stride with both the right and the left leg.)

Repeat the entire combination four times, alternating sides — twice with the right leg and twice with the left.

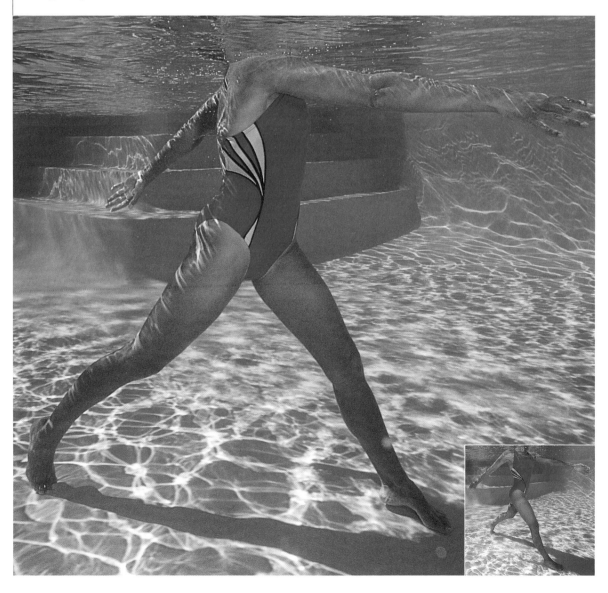

STAR 2

Following Star 1, which combined front kneelifts, kicks, and strides, we now change to side-to-side movements, ending with crossover jacks. This combination gives your quads, abductors, and adductors a great workout. Use your arms as well as your legs – the more you move the more calories you'll burn.

CAUTION Protect your low back by keeping the abdominals contracted when you turn out the leg and when you bring the foot behind the opposite leg.

INTENSITY Increase the intensity by hopping from one foot to the other in the kneelifts and kicks. To work the glutes even harder, keep the leg straight as you lower it to the floor.

2 **SIDE KICK.** As in Step 1, start with a right then a left side kneelift. After the third kneelift, extend the leg into a side kick. Bend and extend twice more (a total of three kicks.) Repeat on the other side, starting with a left side kneelift. Continue for at least eight repetitions.

1 **SIDE KNEELIFT.** Start from neutral position, with the feet hip-width apart and the knees soft. Turn the right hip out and raise the leg in a side kneelift. Repeat to the left, and continue alternating sides for at least eight complete repetitions. (A complete repetition includes a side kneelift on both the right and the left side.) Swing the arms toward the working leg to help balance.

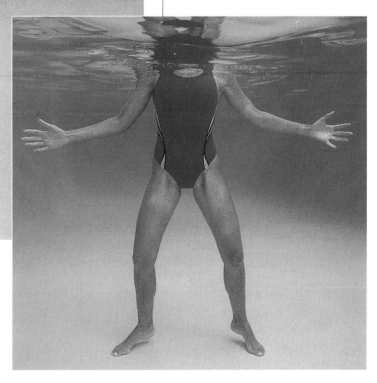

3 CROSSOVER JACK. Bring the leg that has just kicked out (here the right) into a crossover jack, so the working leg is crossed at the ankle in front of the supporting leg. At the same time, cross the arms in front of the body, with the corresponding arm (here the right) in front of the other.

4 OPEN THE JACK. Jump the legs apart, at the same time opening the arms out to the sides. Repeat Steps 3 and 4 four times. Repeat on the other side, crossing the left foot in front of the right and bringing the left arm in front of the right. Continue alternating the crossover for a total of four crossover jacks. Repeat the entire combination, starting with a left side kneelift.

STAR 3

Now that you've got your legs going front and side, you can increase the intensity with water jogging. Here, the working leg comes up behind the body with the knee directly under the hip. Make sure that the hips remain square to the front. After the jogs, tighten up the glutes even more with back kicks and lunges.

CAUTION Be very careful of the low back in this exercise. Lunges and back kicks may cause hyperextension of the back, with subsequent pain. Keep the knees in alignment under the body.

INTENSITY Increase intensity by raising the foot higher on the jogs, by making the back kicks bigger, and by pushing harder with the arms on the lunges.

1 JOG. Start from neutral position, with the feet hip-width apart and the knees soft. Begin jogging, lifting the right foot up behind you while maintaining both knees under the hips. Repeat with the left leg and continue, alternating sides for at least eight complete repetitions. (A complete repetition includes a right and a left jog.) The arms perform complementary movements, moving in opposition to the legs.

2 KNEE FORWARD. As in Step 1, start with a right then a left jog. After the third jog, bring the right knee forward with the knee bent, in preparation for the back kick in Step 3.

Note that the arms are now working in opposition — as the right leg goes forward, the right arm goes back, and vice versa.

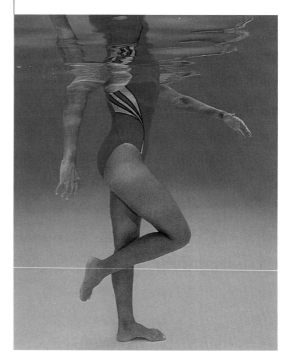

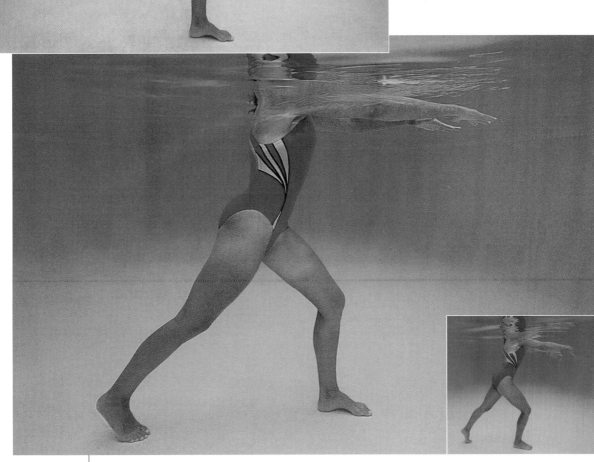

3 BACK KICK. From the knee forward position (Step 2), extend the right leg straight back into a back kick. Repeat this twice for a total of two back kicks, ending with the right knee forward. Repeat on the other side, starting with a left then a right jog. Repeat Steps 2–3 at least four times.

4 BACK LUNGE. After completing the previous sequence, extend and lower the leg to the back. Only the ball of the foot touches the floor. As you lower your foot, bring both arms out in front of the body, parallel to the floor. Return to neutral position, pulling your hands in to rest on your hips. Lunge back with the opposite foot, then return to neutral position. Repeat alternating back lunges for two complete repetitions.

STAR 4

In Star 4, we work further on hip mobility, with a series of open and crossover kneelifts, which require turning the hips in and out as the bent knee crosses in front of the midline. Concentrate on maintaining correct alignment, and avoid rounding your shoulders forward as you move your arm toward the opposite raised leg.

CAUTION Keep the back straight. Do not hunch over or lower your shoulders toward the foot. Maintain the alignment of the hip, knee, and foot.

INTENSITY Increase intensity by hopping from one leg to the other during kneelifts. Keep the hands open, separating the fingers. Use the arms forcefully in opposition to the leg movements.

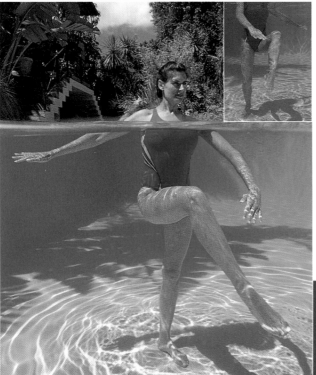

2 DIAGONAL KICK. As in Step 1, start with a right then a left open kneelift. After the third open kneelift, move directly into a diagonal kick that is halfway between a front and a side kick. Repeat to the left, starting with a left open kneelift, and continue for at least four complete repetitions. As the right leg kicks, the arms swing to the left, and vice versa.

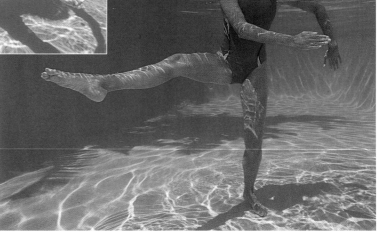

1 OPEN KNEELIFT. Starting from neutral, turn the right hip out and bring your right instep up in front of the body. Repeat to the left, and continue alternating sides for eight complete repetitions. As the right leg lifts, the right arm is out to the side, the left arm toward the foot, and vice versa.

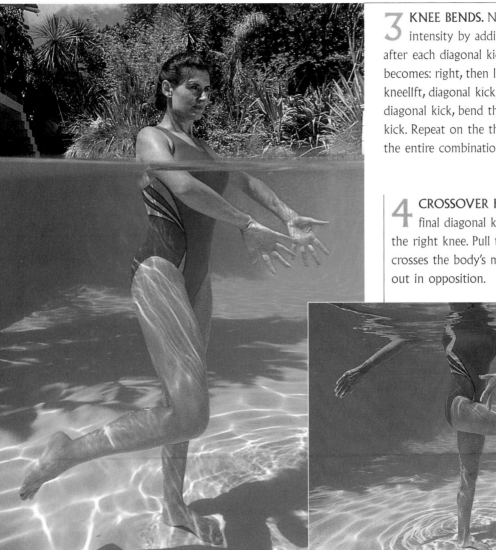

3 **KNEE BENDS.** Now we increase intensity by adding two knee bends after each diagonal kick. The sequence becomes: right, then left, then right open kneellft, diagonal kick, bend the knee, diagonal kick, bend the knee, diagonal kick. Repeat on the the other side. Repeat the entire combination four times.

4 **CROSSOVER KNEELIFT.** After a final diagonal kick in Step 3, bend the right knee. Pull the leg in until it crosses the body's midline. The arms go out in opposition.

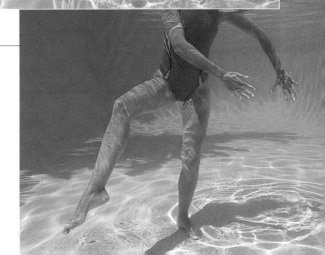

5 **SIDE KNEELIFT.** With the right knee still bent, turn the hip out, in external rotation, into a side kneelift, or as far as you can go. The arms are now out to the left. Repeat Steps 4 and 5 four times.

Repeat the entire combination (Steps 2–5) four times, alternating the side on which you start working. You will feel the mobility of the hip joint increase as you repeat these movements.

STAR 5

In this powerful sequence, we combine hopscotch, side kicks, and rocking horses. Each time you repeat the sequence, you will do it better, bigger, and with more control. On the rocking horses, increase the intensity by traveling forward in the water as you rock, using your arms more forcefully to push the water.

CAUTION When touching the opposite foot with the hand, lean over to the side, lowering the ribs toward the hip. Do not kick higher than is comfortable for you.

INTENSITY Increase intensity by using the arms to contrast the rocking horses – that is, when the front leg goes down, the arms come up, and when the front leg comes up, the arms go down.

2 SIDE KICK. As in Step 1, start with a right and left hopscotch. After the third hopscotch, when the right foot is behind the left knee, extend the right leg into a side kick. Repeat the movement on the other side. Continue alternating sides for at least eight repetitions.

1 HOPSCOTCH. Starting from neutral position, turn the right hip out and bend the right knee so the foot is behind the supporting leg. Try to touch the right foot with the left hand. Repeat with the left leg and continue, alternating sides for at least eight complete repetitions. (A complete repetition includes a hopscotch on both the right and the left side.)

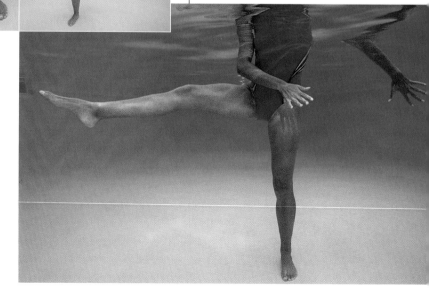

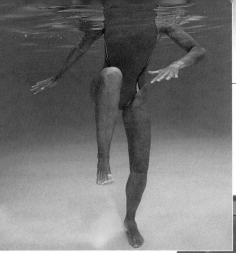

3 **KNEELIFT.** After repeating the combination once more leading with the right leg, pull in the right leg from the side kick to a front kneelift. The arms will help to stabilize the position.

4 **SIDE KICK.** Kick the right leg out to the side. Push the arms out to the opposite side. Repeat Steps 3 and 4, then repeat the entire sequence from Step 1, starting with a left leg lead. Repeat the combination at least four times.

5 **ROCKING HORSES.** After performing the last side kick, turn to face the right and bring the right leg up in a front kneelift in preparation for the rocking horses. Keep the supporting knee bent. Both arms go forward as you turn your body.

6 **ROCKING HORSES.** As you bring the right leg down, lift the left leg back in a jog. Pushing the water with the arms, perform four complete rocking horses. Repeat the combination, starting from the hopscotch (Step 1) with a left leg lead. Repeat the entire combination four times.

STAR 6

After the excitement of Star 5, with its hopscotches, side kicks, and rocking horses, we move into the realm of the front high kicks. This combination will keep you moving and tone your adductor muscles, quads, and glutes. Keep your shoulders square with your hips as you bring the leg across the midline to kick.

CAUTION Respect the hip-knee-foot alignment on the support leg during the crossovers. Do not lock the knee when extending or lowering the leg.

INTENSITY Keep the legs extended as you lower them from the high kicks. Concentrate on the down part of the high kick, not on the up part.

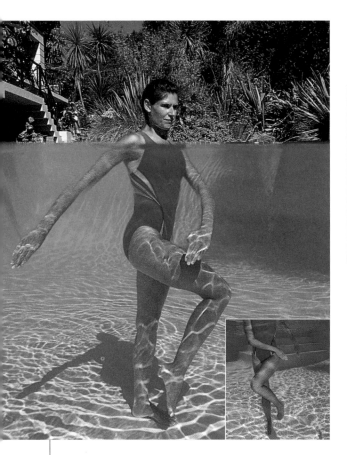

2 CROSSOVER KICK. Start with a right then a left crossover kneelift. After the third kneelift, extend the right leg into a low crossover kick. Repeat on other side, alternating for four repetitions. Begin the combination again, and after the right low crossover kick, add four alternating crossover kicks. Swing the arms to the right as the right leg kicks forward, and vice versa. Repeat on the other side. Repeat the entire combination four times.

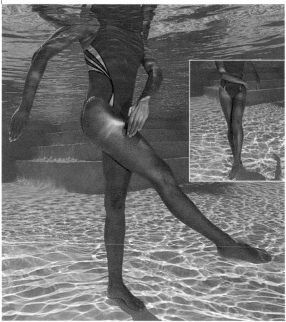

1 CROSSOVER KNEELIFT. Starting from neutral, turn the right hip in, and lift the knee across the midline. Repeat to the left and continue, alternating sides for eight complete repetitions. (A complete repetition includes a crossover kneelift on both the right and the left.) Arms swing to the right as the right leg moves to the left and vice versa.

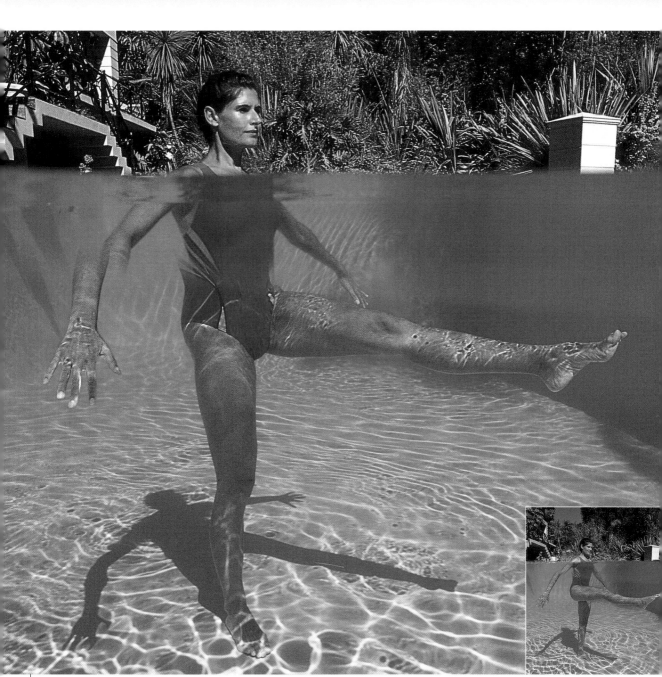

3 **HIGH FRONT KICK.** Repeat from Step 2 and, after the fifth low crossover kick, perform a total of eight high front kicks, alternating legs. Use your hands and arms to push back as you raise your legs for the high kicks. Repeat the complete combination (Steps 1–3) four times, alternating sides. If you wish, turn the body slowly clockwise during the high kicks so that you begin facing obliquely to the left and finish facing obliquely to the right, and vice versa on the other side.

SUPERSTAR

This is a fabulous sequence, providing a great workout and taking your legs in the various directions of the star. Feel the strength in your thighs, the mobility of your hips, and the power in your center as you move your arms with grace and precision. You may even visualize yourself twinkling!

CAUTION Keep the back straight and the abdominals tight to stabilize the core. Lean forward when you perform the back kick, contracting the glutes to control its height. Do not arch the low back.

INTENSITY Keep the hands open and cupped to increase the intensity. Keep the legs straight as you lower them from the high kicks to increase the load on the glutes.

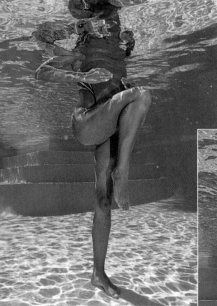

2 FRONT KICK. As in Step 1, start with a right then a left front kneelift. After the third kneelift extend the right leg into a front kick. As you lower the right leg, raise the left leg into a front kneelift then kick to the front. Continue for at least eight repetitions.

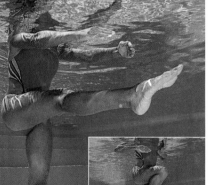

3 SIDEKICK. From the kneelift position, turn the right leg out to the side and extend the leg into a side kick. The sequence now becomes right kneelift, right front kick, right kneelift, right side kick. Repeat on the other side, then alternate sides for at least four complete repetitions.

1 FRONT KNEELIFT. Starting from neutral position, raise the right knee in front of the body. Repeat with the left leg and continue, alternating sides for at least eight repetitions. The elbows are bent and the hands are at rib-height in front of the body.

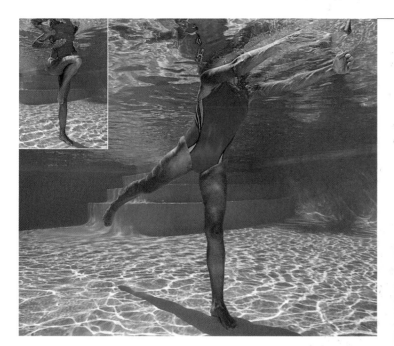

4 **BACK KICK** From the right front kneelift position, extend the right leg into a back kick. Return to the kneelift position and kick the leg to the front. Repeat Steps 2–4 on the other side, starting with a left front kneelift, then perform four complete repetitions, alternating sides.

5 **FRONT HIGH KICK**. Finally, when you lower the right leg, start alternating front high kicks with the left and right legs for a total of four complete repetitions. Repeat the entire combination from the first front kick (Step 2) for at least four complete repetitions, alternating sides.

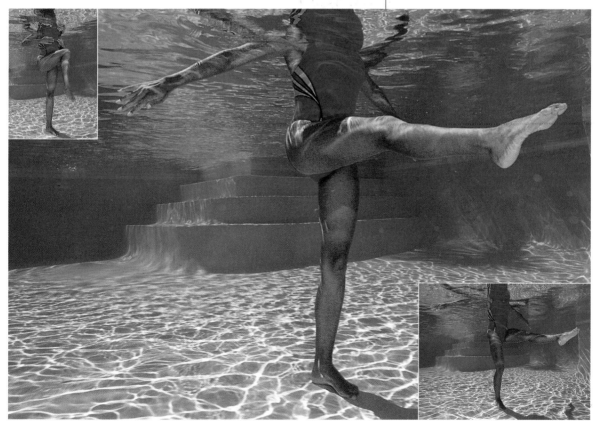

PENDULUM / JUMPING JACK COMBINATION

The hard part In these side-to-side movements, which work the hip abductors and adductors, is bringing the foot down to the ground on the pendulums and together on the jacks. Imagine the legs as being long and powerful as they push through the water.

CAUTION Do not raise the leg so far as to go out of alignment. The higher you raise the leg, the harder you have to work to push it down. Keep the abdominals tight and your core stabilized. Do not lock the knees.

INTENSITY Use the arms forcefully to help you travel on the pendulums and to push you forward and back on the jacks.

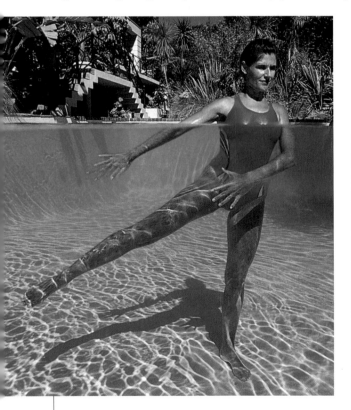

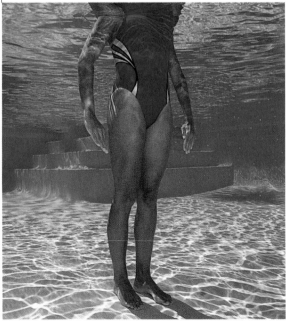

2 NEUTRAL. In Step I, we brought the feet together in neutral position between alternating pendulums. Now repeat same-side pendulums, performing eight with the right leg and eight with the left, bringing the feet together in neutral position between each pendulum.

1 PENDULUM. Starting from neutral position hop onto the left leg and raise the right leg out to the side. Keep the supporting knee soft. The arms push in the same direction as the raised leg. Hop the feet back together then continue, alternating sides for eight complete repetitions. (A complete repetition comprises both a right and a left leg pendulum.)

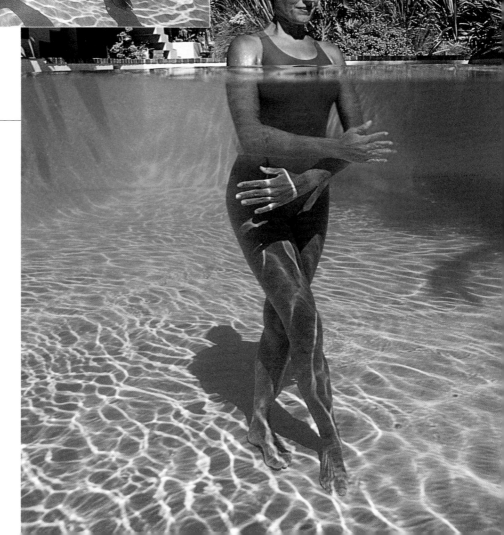

3 JUMPING JACK. After completing the last pendulum, hop and open the legs. Hop again and bring the feet together. Repeat eight jumping jacks. Arms echo the leg movements, opening out to the sides and closing in front of the body. Use the arms to help you travel forward for four jacks and back for four.

4 CROSSOVER JACK.

We now increase the intensity by enlarging the range of motion. Hop, opening both legs as before, but when you hop back, cross the right leg in front of the left and the right arm in front of the left. Hop the legs apart again, and cross the left leg in front as you return. Left arm is in front of right. Repeat eight complete crossover jacks. Repeat the entire sequence (Steps 1–4) four times.

NEFERTITI COMBINATION

This is a fun combination. The Nefertiti pose gives an unusual sensation because the hands are not in opposition with the legs – as your right leg comes forward, the right arm comes forward and vice versa. Everything goes back to normal with the stride.

CAUTION Lift your feet to avoid scraping them on the floor. Keep your back knee directly under your hip in the Nefertiti pose. Keep the abdominals tight when you bring the leg back in the strides.

INTENSITY Increase intensity by lifting the legs in a tuck jump from the neutral or the open position. During the strides, move the arms and legs forcefully in the water.

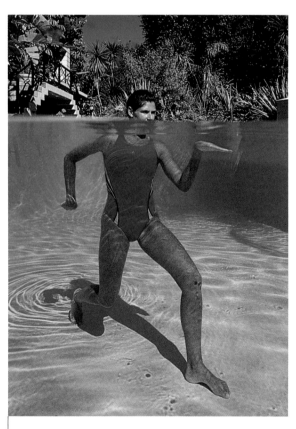

2 RETURN TO CENTER. Swiveling your feet again, return to center with your hands by your sides, palms downward. Bounce twice in this neutral position.

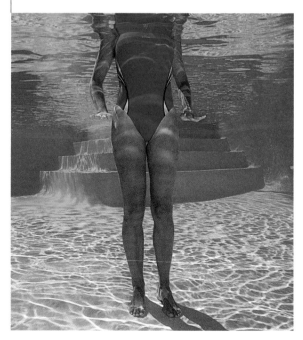

1 SWIVEL LEFT. Start from neutral position, with the feet hip-width apart and the knees soft. Turn your body to face left, swiveling your feet as you turn. Bounce twice in this position. With elbows bent, raise your left arm in front of you, leaving the right arm behind in the Nefertiti pose. Bounce twice in this position.

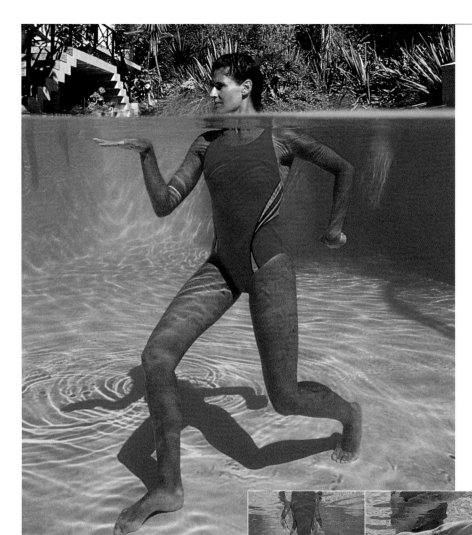

3 **SWIVEL RIGHT.**
Swiveling your feet, turn your body to face right. Raise your right arm in front of you, leaving the left arm behind in the Nefertiti position. Bounce twice. Return to the neutral position and bounce twice. Repeat this combination (Steps 1–3) four times. (A complete repetition includes a left swivel, a bounce, a right swivel, and a bounce.)

4 **STRIDE**. Swiveling the feet again, face to the left. This time the left foot goes forward and the right foot goes back in a stride. The arms are complementary, working in opposition. Perform 16 strides. On the last stride, return to neutral and face forward. Repeat the stride sequence on the other side, turning to the right to begin. Repeat the entire combination (Steps 1–4) at least four times.

DEEP-WATER

COMBINATIONS

Working in deep water eliminates impact and stress on joints. You will need a flotation belt to keep you afloat, but with it, you'll feel as if you are dancing on a cloud and you'll walk out feeling ten feet tall. In deep water, the abdominals must be kept very tight to ensure trunk stability, and you must stabilize your legs vertically by tightening the glutes. Once you're strong enough, you may want to use aquafins and webbed gloves to increase the intensity of the workout. Again, remember to start with a warmup and end with a cooldown (*see pp30–31*).

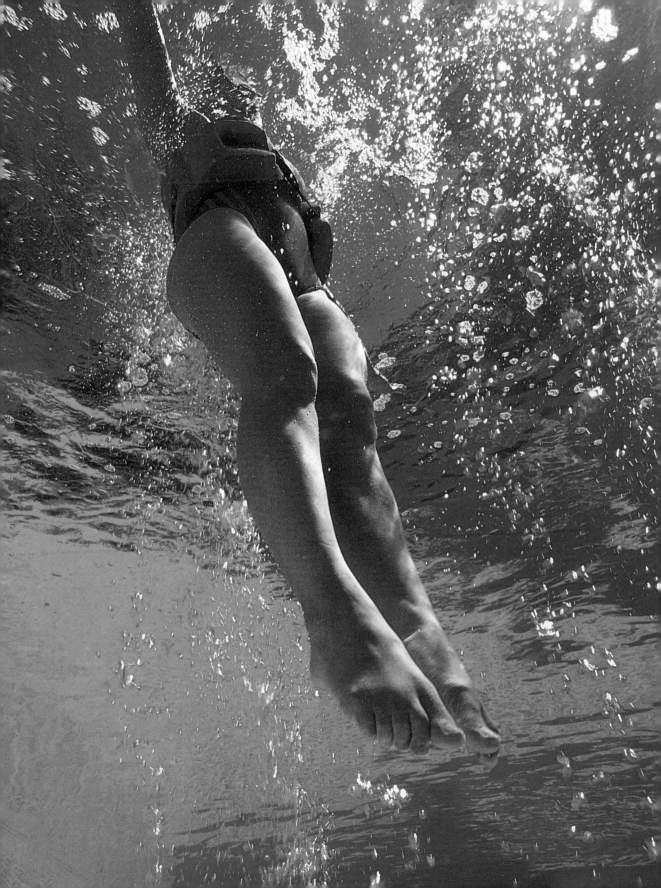

OCTOPUS 1

The Octopus is the deep-water equivalent of the Star combinations, which we practiced in the previous chapter. Despite wearing a flotation belt, you will find it more difficult to control your movements and stay vertical in deep water. It may help to visualize a weight attached to the big toe of the stabilizing leg.

CAUTION Try to keep the back relaxed. Tighten the glutes and the quads to help keep you vertical.

INTENSITY Increase the intensity by lowering the leg forcefully, initiating the movement with the glutes. Stride the arms and legs powerfully, in as large a range of motion as possible.

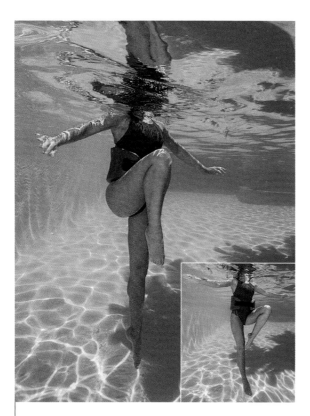

2 KICK. As in Step 1, start with a right then a left kneelift. After the third kneelift, extend the right leg into a front kick. The left leg continues to point to the floor and the arms remain out to the sides, stabilizing your position. Repeat on the other side, starting with a left front kneelift. Continue for eight complete repetitions.

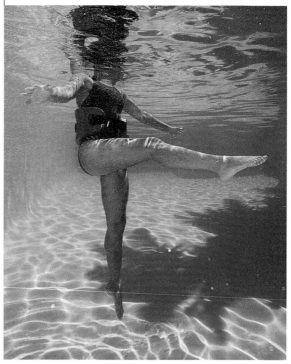

1 KNEELIFTS. Start in neutral position, with both feet pointing straight down. Arms are out to the sides to help stabilize and maintain your position in the pool. Ensure that your body is vertical at all times. Raise the right knee in a front kneelift, then repeat with the left leg. Continue, alternating sides for eight complete repetitions (a complete repetition includes a right and left front kneelift), or as many as you need to maintain your balance.

3 PEDAL FORWARD. Repeat Step 2 and after the right front kick, bend the right knee and start pedaling, leading with the heel. Repeat the pedaling movement twice, then repeat the combination on the other side, starting with a left kneelift. Perform at least eight complete repetitions, alternating sides. Concentrate on maintaining a vertical position in the water as you pedal. The arms remain out to the sides to stabilize your position.

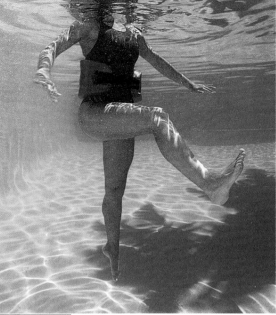

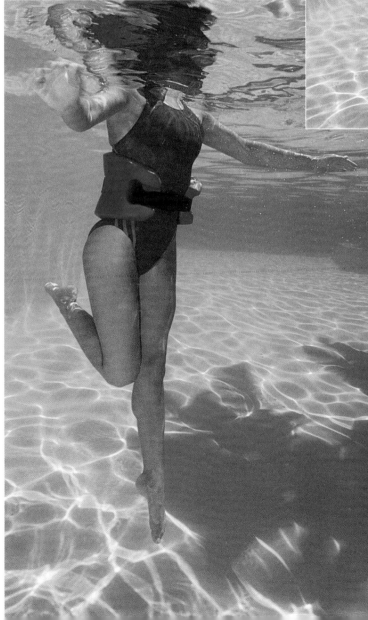

4 PREPARE TO STRIDE. After the last pedal, bring the right leg to the back then bring the left leg forward in a stride. Switch legs and repeat until you have performed eight deep-water strides. The arms work in opposition to the legs. Repeat the entire combination (Steps 1–4), starting with a left front kneelift. Continue for four complete repetitions, alternating sides.

OCTOPUS 2

In deep water, you can move your legs in ways that are not possible in shallow water. We make good use of this here, with some great exercises to increase hip mobility and tone the glutes and thighs. Visualize flattening the abdominals and lengthening the legs as you reach full extension in the kicks and stretches.

CAUTION Hold the abdominals tight to maintain spinal integrity and trunk stabilization. Remember to keep your shoulders back and down and your head up.

INTENSITY Increase intensity by forcefully pushing your legs through the water on the half frogs. Use your arms to help keep you in the same spot in the water as you perform the leg movements.

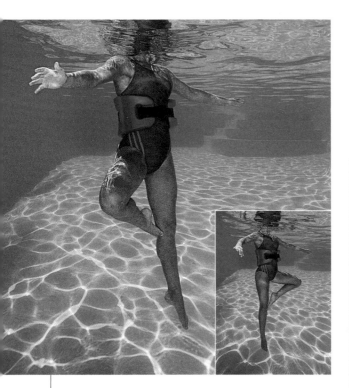

2 SIDE QUAD KICK. As in Step 1, start with a right then a left side kneelift. After the third kneelift, perform a side quad kick. Repeat on the other side, starting with a left side kneelift. Continue for at least eight complete repetitions.

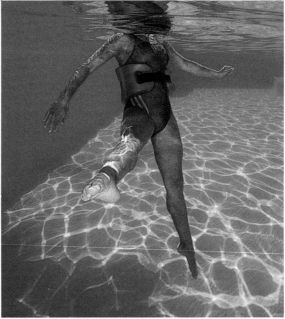

1 SIDE KNEELIFT. Start in neutral position, with both legs pointing straight down to the floor. Turn the right leg out at the hip and raise the knee in a side kneelift. Return to neutral and repeat with the left leg. Continue alternating sides for at least eight complete repetitions, or until you can perform the side kneelifts without arching the low back. Keep the stabilizing leg straight, pointing directly down to the floor. The arms are out to the sides to help keep you stationary in the water.

3 **FROG**. Repeat the combination once more as in Step 2. After the side quad kick, bring both feet in so that the toes touch under the body. We call this the "frog." Keep the glutes very tight in order to keep your knees pointing directly out to the sides.

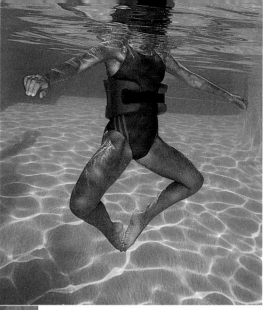

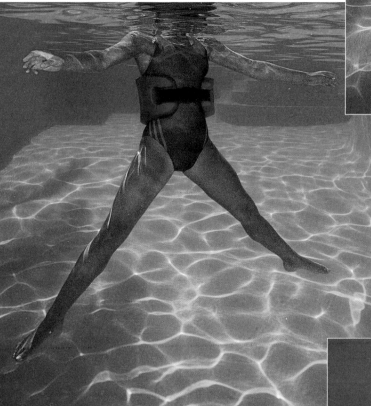

4 **SIDE LEG EXTENSIONS**. From the frog, straighten both legs, keeping the thighs and knees in the same position. Repeat the frog and straighten the legs once more. Repeat the sequence from Step 2, starting with a left side kneelift. Repeat the entire combination four times, alternating sides.

5 **HALF FROGS**. Repeat Step 4, beginning the sequence with a right side kneelift. After the last frog extension, leave the right leg extended and flex the left knee, bringing the foot under the body in a "half frog." Repeat the half frogs, alternating sides for four complete repetitions. Repeat this combination, starting with a left side kneelift. Perform the complete combination (Steps 1–5) at least four times, alternating sides.

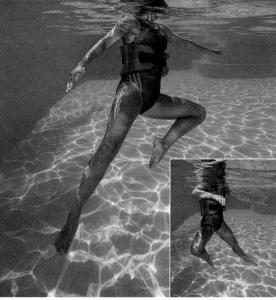

OCTOPUS 3

This combination is a real challenge. You will be working on your hip mobility in Octopus 3, and discovering parts of your anatomy that you didn't know you had. As you perform the exercise, try visualizing yourself as vertical while you trace a big circle around your body with your pointed toes.

CAUTION Keep your abdominal muscles contracted throughout this exercise in order to stabilize the trunk. When the abdominal muscles are contracted, the back muscles should be relaxed.

INTENSITY This exercise is not intended so much for intensity as for mobility and control. Think big as you circle the legs.

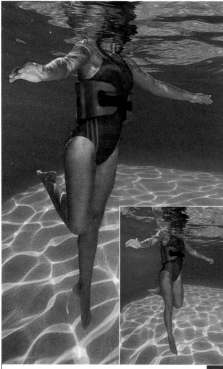

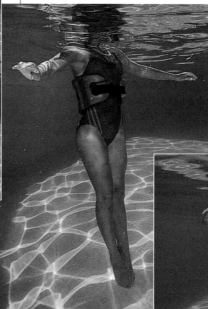

2 NEUTRAL After the third jog, extend the legs down to neutral. Tighten your glutes and abdominals to maintain posture, balance, and vertical position.

3 BEND KNEES. Bend both knees, bringing your legs up behind you in a "kneeling" position. Knees point directly to the pool floor. Repeat twice, straightening the legs after each bend. Repeat Steps 1–3 four times, alternating sides.

1 JOG. Start in neutral position, with both feet pointing down. Bend the right knee, bringing the leg up behind the thigh. Knees are under the body. Repeat with the left leg. Continue, alternating sides, for at least eight repetitions or until you can do the jogs and maintain your vertical position.

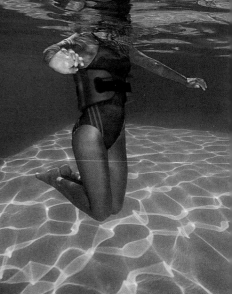

4 **BEND AND TUCK**. Bend the legs behind you once more, as in Step 3, then pull them up in front of the body. Keep the legs together and continue pointing the feet down toward the pool floor. Contract the abdominals to keep the hips stabilized. Use your arms to stabilize your position in the water.

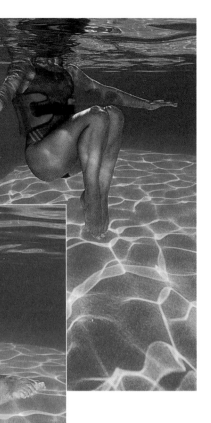

5 **EXTEND LEGS**. After the tuck, extend your legs straight out in front of you as if you were seated. Concentrate on keeping your upper body upright in the water.

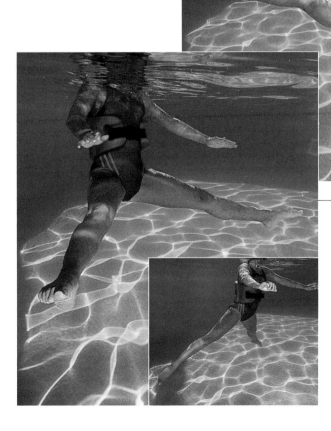

6 **CIRCLE LEGS**. Continuing from Step 5, separate the legs and begin circling the legs: right leg to the right and left leg to the left. Trace an imaginary circle around the body with the legs, starting from the front until they come back together behind your body. Do not arch the low back when the legs are behind the body.

Repeat the combination from Step 1, starting with a left leg jog. Repeat the entire combination four times, alternating sides.

OCTOPUS 4

This part of the Octopus sequence focuses on the quadriceps, hamstrings, and gluteals. Think about your gluteal muscles as you contract them – visualize them tightening, lifting with the buoyancy of the water, and overcoming gravity. As I tell my students, "If you don't think about your glutes, no one else will!"

CAUTION Be careful to maintain proper alignment between the hip, knee, and foot on the leg kicks and circles.

INTENSITY To increase intensity, use your arms in large range of motion movements on the knee-lifts. Use the force of the kick, not your arms, to propel your body around the 360° turn. You should feel it in your hamstrings.

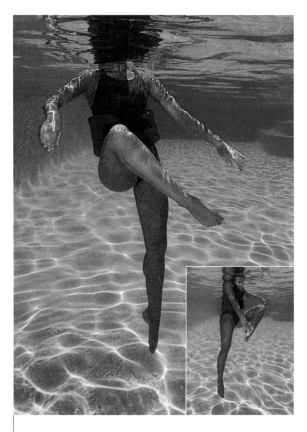

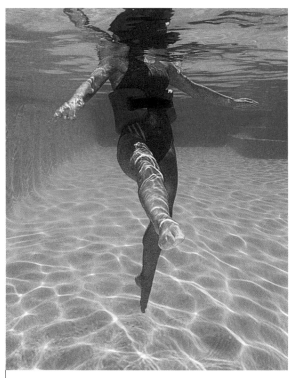

1 KNEELIFTS. Start in neutral position, with both feet pointing straight down. Keeping the back straight, turn the right leg out at the hip, and raise it in an open kneelift. Try to touch the instep of the raised foot with the opposite hand, without curving your back. As you lower the right leg, raise the left leg in an open kneelift. Continue for at least eight complete repetitions, alternating sides.

2 KICKS AND LEG CIRCLES. As in Step 1, start with a right and a left open kneelift. After the third kneelift, extend the leg into a diagonal kick. Bend the knee and circle the leg twice, counter-clockwise. As you lower the right leg, raise the left leg to repeat the combination on the other side, starting with a left open kneelift. Circle the left leg clockwise. Repeat the entire sequence four times.

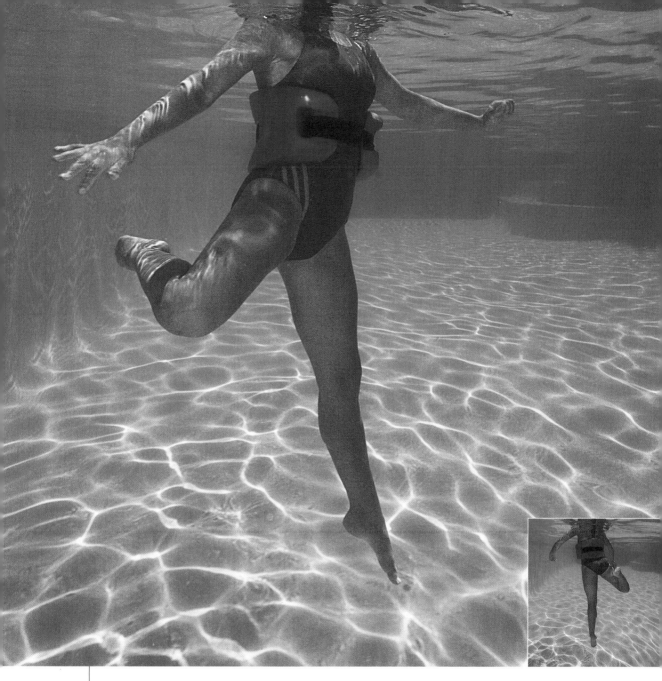

3 **KICK AND TURN**. Start once more as in Step 2, with a right leg lead. At the end of the leg circles, leave the right leg raised, but turn it inward so the foot points to the back. Contracting the gluteus, flex and extend the leg, kicking eight times to turn the body around 360°. If you are working to music, try to complete the turn in 16 beats. As you lower the right leg, raise the left leg to begin the sequence on the other side with an open kneelift. Repeat the entire combination (Steps 2–3) four times, alternating between a right leg lead and a left leg lead.

OCTOPUS 5

We complete the Octopus sequence with crossover kneelifts and kicks. Try to keep your upper body still as the lower body twists into the crossovers. Feel your abdominals tighten to keep your back lengthened and protected. As you stride, enjoy the sensation of the water massaging your thighs and your legs. Heavenly!

CAUTION If you suffer from back pain, be very careful when doing the twist — keep the back straight and in proper alignment. If twisting is inappropriate, you may do the crossover kneelift without twisting the trunk, but by having just the knee cross the midline.

INTENSITY To increase intensity, stride with powerful arm and leg movements.

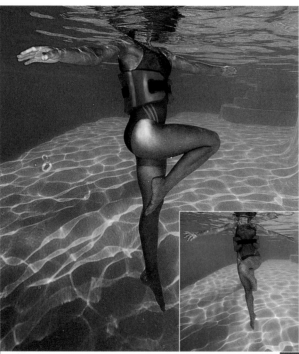

2 CROSSOVER KICK. As in Step 1, start with a right then a left crossover kneelift. After the third kneelift, extend the right leg into a crossover kick. As you lower the right leg, raise the left leg in a crossover kneelift. Perform at least eight complete repetitions, alternating sides. You will feel your quadriceps and adductor muscles contract and tighten up as you perform the crossover kicks.

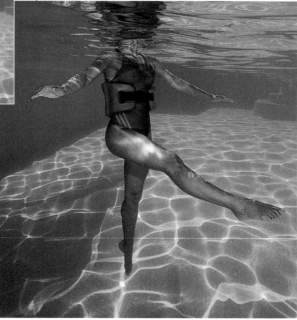

1 CROSSOVER KNEELIFTS. Start in neutral position, with both legs pointing down to the floor. Turn the right hip in, bend the knee, and raise the leg in a crossover kneelift. Push the right leg back to neutral while raising the left leg in a crossover kneelift. Continue, alternating sides for at least eight complete repetitions, or until you can maintain perfect vertical alignment while performing the crossover kneelifts. Arms are out to the sides to help maintain the position of the upper body.

3 BEND KNEE. When you have perfected the cross-over kneelifts and kicks, bend and extend the leg twice. When you bring the leg back and bend the knee, contract the glutes to pull the thigh back. The foot will be brought up towards the glutes.

4 HIGH KICK. From the jog position (Step 3), straighten the right leg and bring it forward into a high crossover kick. Repeat twice, then lower the right leg and repeat the sequence (Steps 3–4), starting with a left crossover kneelift. Repeat the complete combination 4–8 times, alternating sides.

5 STRIDES. To finish this combination, add on eight strides, alternating lead legs. Keep the legs straight and the knees soft. Make the strides as big as possible, as if you were performing splits.

Repeat the 16 movements of the combination, starting with a left crossover kneelift (Step 2). Continue for four complete repetitions, alternating sides.

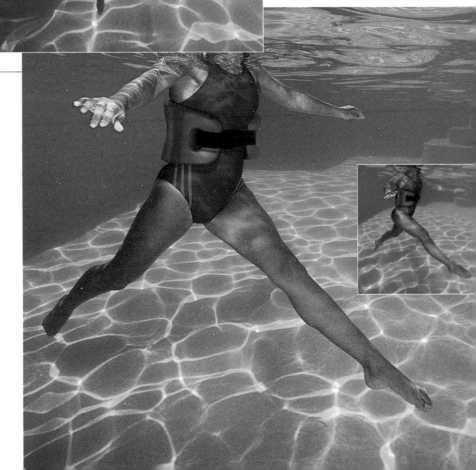

JUMPING JACK COMBINATION

After the directional variety of the Octopus sequences, you'll have no trouble with the next combination. Aside from being an excellent exercise for hip mobility, it is one of the best exercises for the inner and outer thighs, toning and stretching both the abductor and the adductor muscle groups (*see pp102–103*).

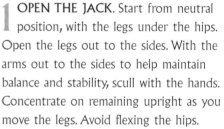

CAUTION Avoid over-contracting the back muscles as you try to remain vertical. Instead, contract the abdominals and keep the low back muscles relaxed.

INTENSITY Increase intensity in the jacks by using the arms with the legs instead of keeping them still, and by pushing the arms and legs forcefully through the water on the bigger jacks.

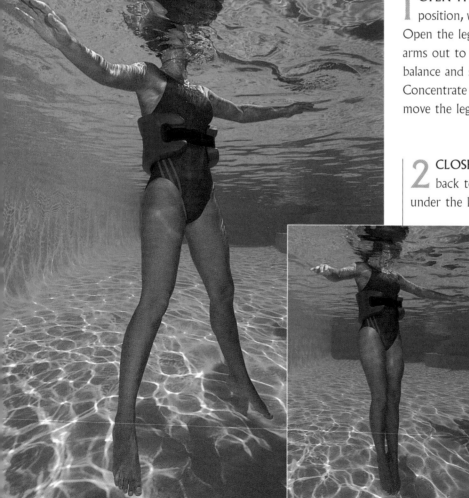

1 **OPEN THE JACK.** Start from neutral position, with the legs under the hips. Open the legs out to the sides. With the arms out to the sides to help maintain balance and stability, scull with the hands. Concentrate on remaining upright as you move the legs. Avoid flexing the hips.

2 **CLOSE THE JACK.** Pull your legs back together, keeping them vertical under the body by holding the glutes and abdominals tight and pointing the feet straight down to the floor. The arms remain out to the sides at chest to shoulder height to help maintain your position in the pool. Repeat the jacks at least eight times, or until you can remain stationary in the pool as you perform them.

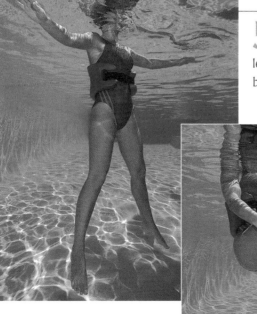

3 **INCREASE THE STRETCH.** Strengthen your outer thighs and increase the stretch on the inner thighs by extending the range of motion of your jacks. Open your legs even wider, while staying perfectly upright in the water. Keep the legs in line with the body.

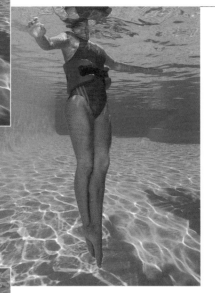

4 **CROSSOVER JACKS.** Now close the jack by bringing the left foot in front of the right, crossing at the ankle. Immediately cross left over right, then right over left. Open the jack and cross three times, now leading with the left foot. Continue alternating the front foot for four crossover jack sequences.

5 **OPEN JACKS** Separate the legs again in preparation for the deep-water hip-hop jack (*see p45*). As you extend the legs, try to get a good stretch through the front of the body, in contrast to the closed position of the hip-hop jack.

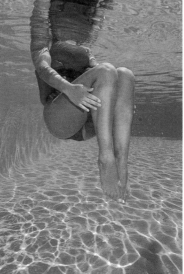

6 **HIP-HOP JACK.** After opening the jack, pull the legs into a tuck under or in front of the body. Contract the abdominals during the tuck to stretch out and relax the low back. The arms pull in to help you tuck. Repeat the deep-water hip-hop jack eight times.

Repeat the entire combination, including four jacks, four crossover jacks, and four hip-hop jacks, for a total of four repetitions.

STRIDE AND CROSS-COUNTRY SKI

This simple combination can be used as a transition between combinations. It is similar to the Jumping Jack combination (*see pp82–83*), but works from front to back, rather than side-to-side, toning the glutes and giving a great stretch to the hip flexors.

CAUTION Be careful not to arch the low back when you extend the leg to the back. Keep the abdominals contracted to protect the lumbar spine.

INTENSITY You can increase the intensity on this combination by increasing the range of motion on both the strides and the circles.

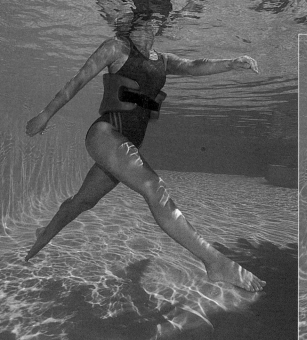

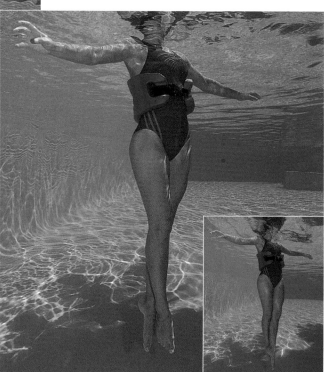

1 STRIDE. Perform 16 alternating strides, starting with the right leg forward. The arms are complementary, so the left arm is forward when the right leg is forward, and vice versa. Make sure that the upper body is upright in the water and that both legs extend an equal distance from the center.

2 CIRCLE FEET. After the last stride, repeat once more with the right leg forward. Come to neutral position with crossed ankles, right foot in front of left. Circle the feet, bringing the left foot in front of the right, then circle again, returning to the original position with the right foot in front of the left. While performing these movements, keep your arms out to the sides to help keep you in an upright position.

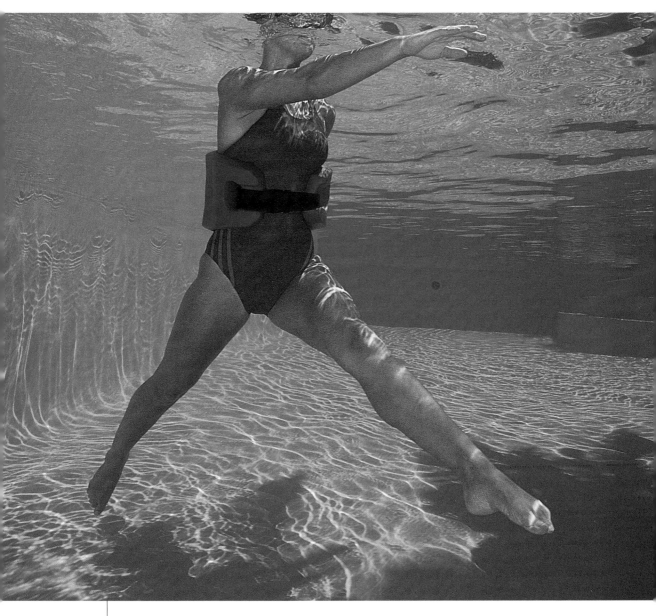

3 STRIDE. Starting with the left leg forward, stride then return to neutral with the ankles crossed, left foot in front of the right. Circle the feet so that the ankles are crossed with the right foot in front, then circle again so the left foot is once more in front. Repeat the entire combination (Steps 1–3) four times, alternating the leading leg.

If you wish to use this as a transitional move, on the last repetition, instead of crossing the ankles, simply unite the feet in neutral position. From here you can go on to any of the other combinations.

ONE-LEGGED KICK AND TURN

You won't find it easy to remain vertical while performing these kicks and turns in deep water – you will have to concentrate on your abdominals to help stabilize you. The secret to staying upright is to point the support leg directly downward.

CAUTION Be careful not to arch the low back when extending the leg back or to the side. Keep the abdominals tight at all times.

INTENSITY Flex and extend the leg twice during the four counts of the hip flexion and extension, increasing the range of motion, and push the abducted leg through the water vigorously to increase acceleration prior to the turn.

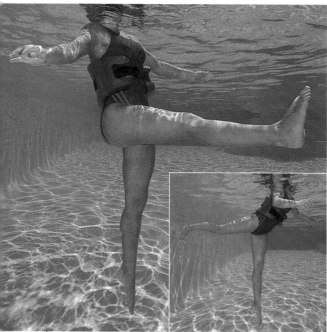

2 SIDE KICK. Repeat the front and back kicks twice more, then raise the right leg in a front high kick. Pull in the leg and take it directly out to the side. Bend and extend the leg in the side kick position. Pull the leg in and return to neutral position. Perform a tiny tuck jump, bending and extending both legs. Repeat the sequence with the left leg. Repeat the combination at least four times.

1 HIGH KICKS Raise the right leg in a front high kick. Arms are out to the sides to stabilize you. Bend and extend the knee, keeping the leg in a high kick. Bend the knee, pull in the leg, and extend it to the back in a back kick. Bend and extend the knee, maintaining the back kick position. Repeat the front and back kick at least eight times, then repeat with the left leg.

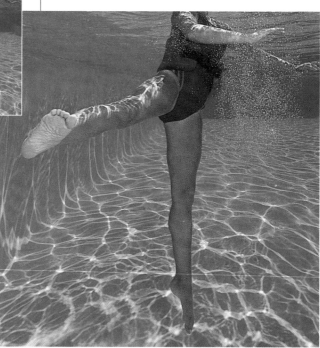

3 START THE TURN. After the last side kick with the right leg, bring the leg in to neutral, crossing the right foot behind the left to begin a 360° clockwise turn. Your arms will help you during the turn, but they should neither initiate the movement nor push the water.

4 CONTINUE TURNING. During the turn, your legs will uncross, so that by 180°, when you are facing in the opposite direction of where you started, your feet will be parallel to each other, under the hips. Try it out on land, to see how it works.

5 COMPLETE TURN. Continue turning until your left leg is crossed behind the right and you are facing forward once again. Then bring the left leg forward in a high kick and repeat the combination on the other side. Repeat the entire combination (Steps 2–5) four times.

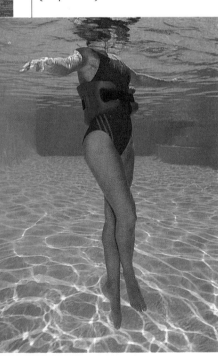

HIGH KICK COMBINATION

Here is another enjoyable combination of high kicks and strides. The large movements will enhance hip mobility and force you to use your abdominal muscles to help stabilize the trunk. The turn is the fun part, making you feel that you can even perform splits!

CAUTION When extending the leg to the back during the 180° turn, be careful not to hyperextend the low back. Keep the abdominals tight and the support leg pointed downward.

INTENSITY Increase the intensity by increasing the range of motion in both the high kicks and the strides.

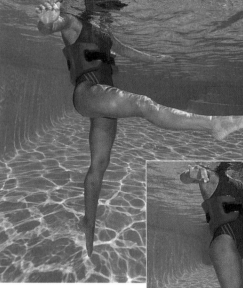

3 FRONT HIGH KICK. Raise the left leg in a front high kick. The arms are still out to the sides and the supporting leg points directly down to the pool floor to help keep you vertical in the water. Bring the leg back to neutral.

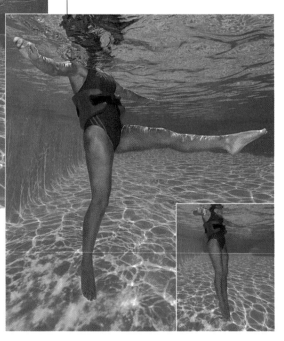

1 FRONT HIGH KICK. Start from neutral position, with both feet pointing down. Working at half-water tempo (*see p25*), raise the right leg in a front high kick. Keep the left leg pointing down to help maintain your upright position. Arms are out to the sides and shoulders are down and back.

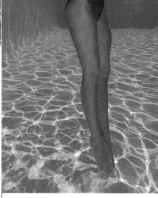

2 NEUTRAL. Bring the right leg back to neutral. Both feet now point to the pool floor. Contract the abdominals to help stabilize the trunk.

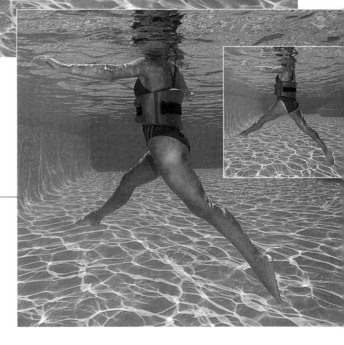

4 **KICK AND TURN**. Working at water tempo (*see p25*), raise the right leg in a high kick. As you lower the right leg, raise the left leg in a high kick. Repeat on the right, but leave the right leg raised. Turn 180° to the left so you are facing back and the right leg now extends to the back.

5 **STRIDE**. From this position, bring the right leg forward and stride for eight repetitions. The arms complement the leg movements. On the last stride, bring the legs back into center and repeat the combination (Steps 1–5) on the opposite side, starting with a half-water tempo high kick with the left leg. Repeat the entire combination four times.

MUSCLE-TONING
EXERCISES

In aquafitness, we have the best possible environment for toning and
stretching every muscle in the body — the water itself. We have
already seen how water works (*see pp10–11*) and identified the major
muscle groups in the human body (*see pp14–15*). Now it's time to start
working them. We'll also look at the equipment you can use to
overload the muscle groups, but with or without such aids,
water is the best possible equipment you can use. Perform
these exercises in chest- to shoulder-depth water, with the legs
in one of the stabilizing positions (*see p23*).

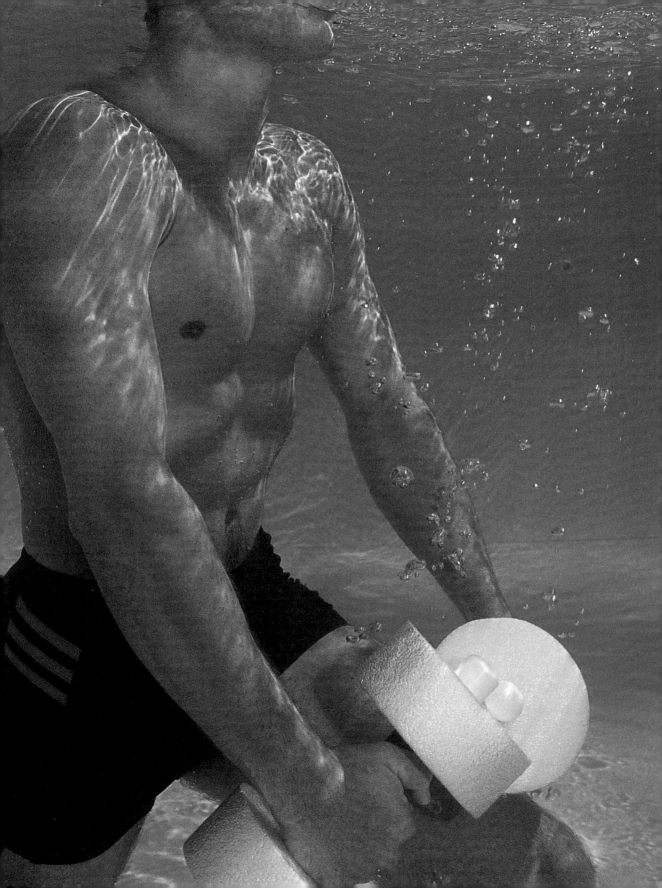

UPPER ARM MUSCLES

These exercises will tone and sculpt the biceps and triceps – the muscles at the front and back of the upper arm, which are responsible for pulling and pushing movements, respectively. The two muscles work in opposition, so as you do the exercises you will be working both. If you exercise them regularly, you can wave goodbye to flabby arms.

CURLS AND KICKBACKS

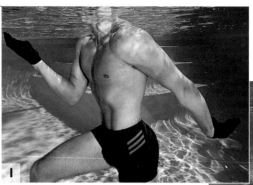

Wearing webbed gloves, start with both arms by your sides. Raise the right arm, bending the elbow and turning the hand so the palm faces you. Extend the left arm back with the elbow straight, palm facing back **1**. Do not lock the elbow. Change arms, raising the left and extending the right **2**. Start with four sets of eight repetitions. (Each repetition includes a right then a left arm forward.) This exercise can also be performed bilaterally.

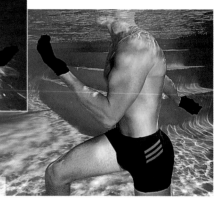

TRICEPS EXTENSIONS

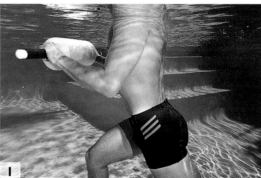

Hold the kickroller or other buoyant equipment in front of you, keeping it under water. Keep your feet rooted to the floor. Your elbows remain close to the body and the shoulders are back and down **1**. Exhaling, lower the kickroller down toward the floor **2**. Slowly allow the kickroller to rise to the initial position, controlling the return with the triceps. Start with two sets of eight repetitions. (Each repetition includes a movement away from the body and a movement toward it.)

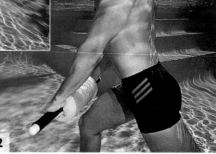

TRICEPS KICKBACKS

Fold a latex band over your right hand and grasp the two ends with the left. The hands will be about 8 in (20 cm) apart, keeping the band in constant tension **1**.

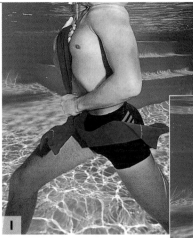

Place your right hand on your chest and, keeping the left elbow near the body, pull the two ends of the band with your left hand, extending the arm backward **2**. Slowly return to the initial position, controlling the elasticity of the band with the tricep. Start with two sets of eight repetitions, then repeat the exercise with the right arm.

PULL-INS AND PUSH-OUTS

Standing in the lunge stabilizing position, hold the closed chain disk by the straps, directly in front of the abdomen. The elbows are bent and close to the body **1**.

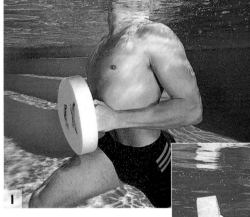

Exhale and push the closed chain disk to the front, away from the body, extending the arms **2**. Keep the shoulders back and down.

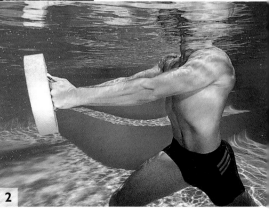

From the extended position, pull the disk back to the original position, controlling the return by contracting the biceps muscles. Start with three sets of eight repetitions.

In this exercise, we are using the closed chain disk mainly for the drag resistance caused by its surface area, but many other muscles will also be working.

CHEST, SHOULDERS, AND UPPER BACK

We now move to the upper body to work the chest muscles (pectorals), those on the front and back of the shoulders (anterior and posterior deltoids), and on the upper back (trapezius and rhomboids). For the best results, keep your shoulders back and down and your elbows soft. Lead with the chest – it's great for posture and self-confidence.

CROSSOVERS AND PULL-BACKS

Start with your arms extended in front of the body with the hands crossed. Open the hands to increase drag resistance **1**.

Keeping the shoulders back and down, pull the extended arms out and back at shoulder height **2**. Hold the position, feeling the stretch in the chest and front shoulder as you contract the traps and rhomboids. Return to the initial position by pulling your arms forward until the hands cross. Keep your shoulders lowered and your head in alignment with the spine. Start with four sets of eight repetitions.

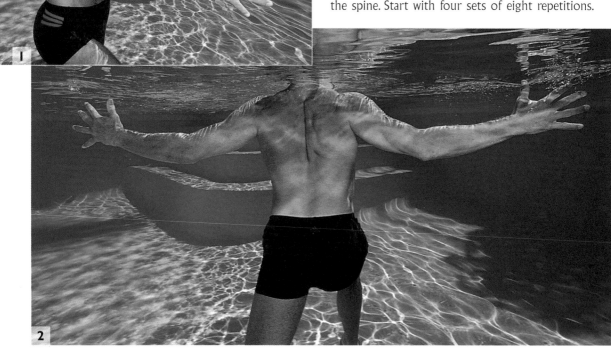

CROSSOVERS WITH LATEX BAND

Pass the band behind the back and under your arms. Holding one end in each hand, and keeping the band under tension, extend the arms out to the sides **1**. Shoulders are back and down.

Pull the arms in toward each other horizontally, stretching the band behind the back and increasing its resistance until the forearms cross **2**.

In this position, you can pulse or make further small contractions of the pecs before bringing the arms back to the initial position. Resisting the pull of the band, control the return of the arms by contracting the pecs. Start with four sets of eight repetitions.

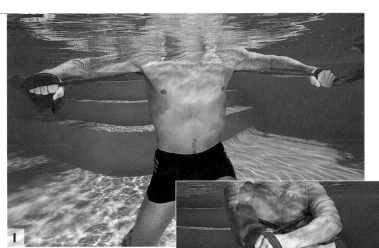

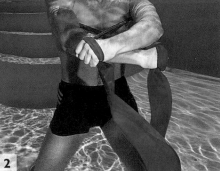

FLOATING PUSH-UPS

Holding the kickroller at chest level, float face-down in the water **1**. Elbows are bent and close to the sides. Keep your abdominals contracted to avoid arching the low back. If you have difficulty keeping your legs up, place a buoyant "noodle" under the ankles until your gluteals are strong enough to keep them straight and floating.

Straightening your arms, push the kickroller down toward the floor in a push-up-type move **2**. Bring the arms back to their original position, controlling the upward thrust of buoyancy by contracting the pecs. Start with two sets of eight repetitions.

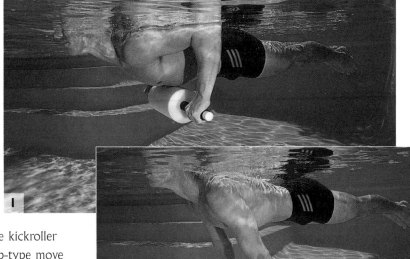

SHOULDER AND BACK MUSCLES

Now let's look at the shoulder muscles (the deltoids) and the opposing large flat muscles of the central back (the latissimus dorsi). The delts are responsible for any action that moves the arm at the shoulder, while any action that brings the arm back down to neutral position or behind the body is effected by the lats. You will feel both sets of muscles working when you perform these exercises, which will increase shoulder mobility.

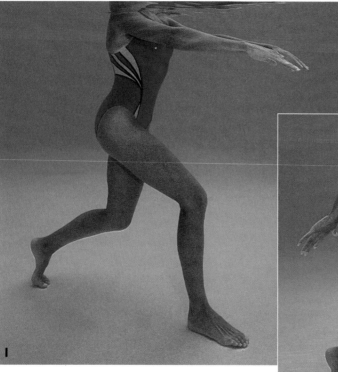

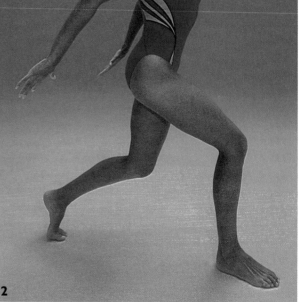

FRONT SHOULDER RAISES AND PRESS-BACKS

Tighten the abdominals and stabilize the trunk. Pull the arms up in front of the body to shoulder height. Hands are flat against the water's resistance, increasing intensity on the anterior deltoid **1**.

Cup the hands and pull the arms down and back, working the lats **2**. Arms are close to the trunk, palms facing back. Shoulders are back and down, and the back is in neutral position. Don't bring the head and shoulders forward in order to raise the arms higher to the back. Start with four sets of eight repetitions.

SHOULDER RAISES AND PULL-DOWNS

For this exercise, wear webbed gloves or aquafins to increase drag resistance. With your shoulders under the water's surface, stand in the lunge stabilizing position as before. Tighten the abdominals and stabilize the trunk. Shoulders are back and down. Bring the arms out to the sides at shoulder height, opening the hands to maximize the drag resistance of the webbed gloves on the medial deltoids **1**.

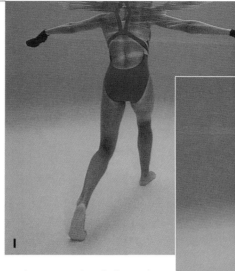

Cup the hands, leaving the fingers spread apart, and pull the arms down and back behind the body until the wrists cross **2**. Do not bring the head and shoulders forward in order to cross the arms further at the back. The head should be in perfect alignment with the spine. Start with four sets of eight repetitions.

PULL-DOWNS WITH BUOYANT EQUIPMENT

This exercise has movements similar to those above, but uses buoyant instead of drag equipment. Because of the equipment's tendency to float, just holding it under water works the lats.

With your shoulders under the water, stand in the lunge stabilizing position as before. Keep the shoulders back and down and hold the handbars out to the sides at shoulder height **1**.

Slowly contracting the lats, bring the arms down and behind the body

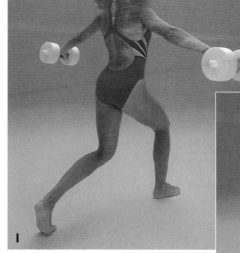

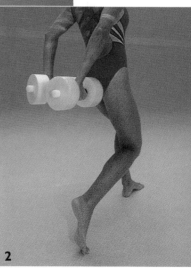

2. You will reach the peak of the contraction when the handbars meet. Release the contraction and return to the starting position, controlling the handbars' buoyant tendency by maintaining the tension in the lats. The deltoids will not be working on this exercise because the buoyancy of the handbars helps to raise the arms. Start with two sets of eight repetitions.

ABDOMINALS AND BACK MUSCLES

The following exercises are great for working the abdominals and the opposing muscle group, the erector spinae. They improve posture and prevent low back pain. The first three can also be done on land. Breathing is the key to success: as you exhale, flatten the abdomen on the contraction; as you inhale, expand the abdomen on the extension.

ABDOMINAL CRUNCHES

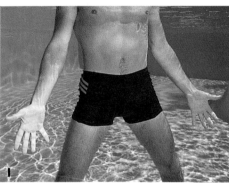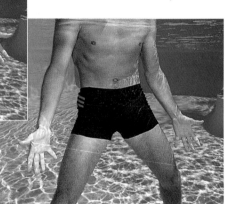

Stand with the legs hip-width apart, arms by your sides. Inhale, expanding the lungs and abdominal cavity **1**.

Exhale, contracting the abdominals and tilting the pelvis up toward the ribs **2**. Feel the vertebrae in your back elongate. Now, inhaling, release the abdominals and return to the original position. Start with four sets of eight consecutive repetitions.

UPPER BODY TWISTS

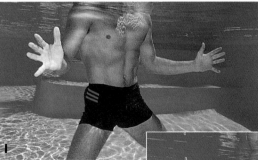

Stand with the feet in a wide stance. Arms are out to the sides. Elbows are bent, near the body. The hands are open. Exhale, contracting the abdominals as above **1**.

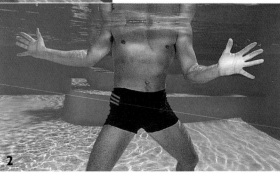

Keeping the lower body in the same position, continue exhaling and rotate the upper body to the right until the shoulders are at a 90° angle to the hips **2**. Inhale and return to the original position. Extend the spine. Repeat, turning in the opposite direction. Start with two sets of eight repetitions. (Each repetition includes a right and a left twist.)

LOWER BODY TWISTS

With the feet in a wide stance, hold the arms out to the sides, elbows bent and near the body. Hands are open. As you exhale, contract the abdominals as before **1**.

Without moving the upper body, continue exhaling and raise the heels, turning them to the right so the hips are at a 90° angle to the shoulders **2**. Inhale and rotate the lower body back to the original position. Finish inhaling as you extend the spine. Repeat the entire exercise in the other direction. Start with two sets of eight repetitions. (Each repetition includes a twist to both the right and the left.)

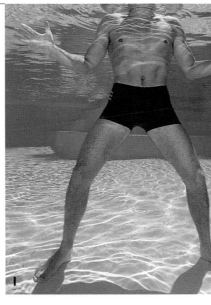

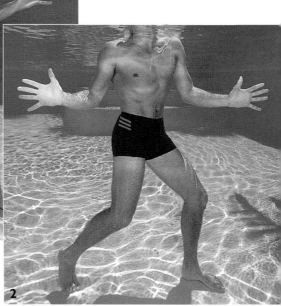

SIDE CRUNCHES

Stand in the stabilizing position of your choice. With the right arm straight, hold a kickroller under the water, in front and slightly to the side of the thigh **1**. Keep the wrist in alignment with the forearm.

Start the exercise with an abdominal crunch (*opposite*) then, exhaling, push the kickroller down. As you do so, pull your right shoulder down toward your right hip **2**.

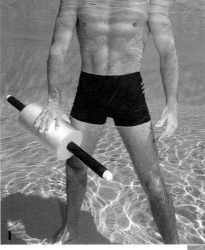

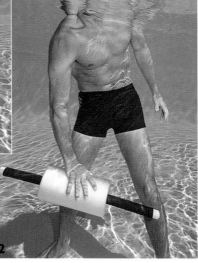

Return to the original position, controlling the upward thrust of buoyancy on the kickroller. Start with two sets of eight repetitions on the right side, then change sides and repeat for two sets of eight repetitions on the left.

ABDOMINALS AND BACK MUSCLES

These deep-water exercises will improve your trunk stability as well as work your abdominal muscles. Unlike doing abdominal exercises on land, there is no floor here to depend upon, and you must find the strength in yourself. Working in deep water without a flotation belt, these exercises are suitable only for those who can swim.

FLOATING REVERSE CURLS

Holding a handbar in each hand or, if you have shoulder problems, under the biceps/triceps muscles, hang in an erect posture with the knees bent, directly under the hips **1**.

Exhaling, tilt the pelvis by contracting the abdominals The thighs come forward **2**. Release the contraction slowly and return to the original position. Start with four sets of eight repetitions.

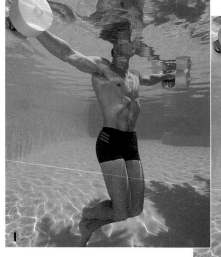
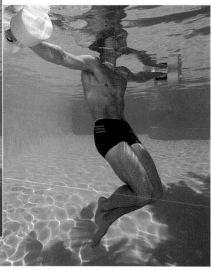

FLOATING CRUNCHES

With a buoyant woggle or noodle placed under the arms and shoulders and another one under the ankles, float on your back **1**. Ensure that you keep your neck relaxed as you float.

As you exhale, contract the abdominals and tilt the pelvis **2**. The hips will tilt as a result of the contraction, stretching the spine. Do not pull in the legs. Inhale and release the contraction, slowly returning to the original position. Start with four sets of eight repetitions.

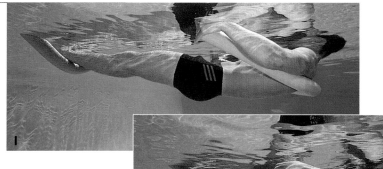
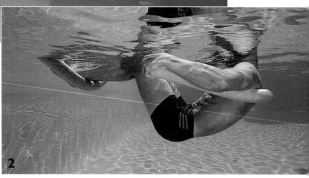

FLOATING TWISTS

Sit on a closed chain disk, with your outstretched arms kept afloat by a handbar in each hand. Keeping the shoulders back and down, maintain an erect posture **1**. Tilt the pelvis by contracting the abdominals. Exhale and twist the lower body to the right until the hips are at 90° to the

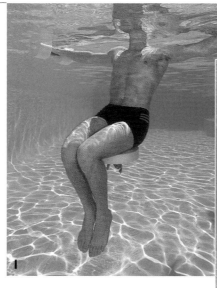

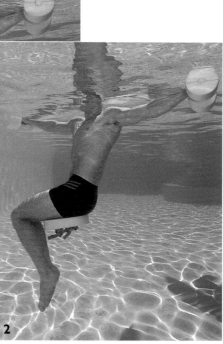

shoulders **2**. Inhale and return to center. Exhaling, repeat the exercise either on the same side or on alternate sides. Start with two sets of eight repetitions on each side.

FLOATING SIDE CRUNCHES

Place the woggle under the arms and behind the back. Hold a handbar in each outstretched hand. The body is upright in the water, the shoulders back and down **1**.

Exhaling, tilt the pelvis by contracting the abdominals, then pull the right hip up toward the right ribs **2**. The left side

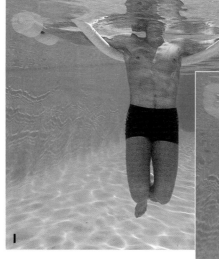

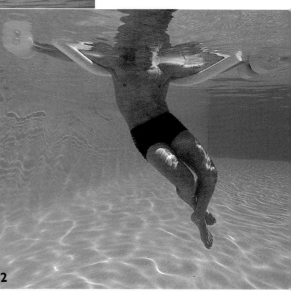

of the body will be stretched as the right side is pulled into a reverse lateral crunch. Inhale and release the contraction, extending the back muscles and relaxing the spine. Repeat this exercise either on the same side or on alternate sides. Start with two sets of eight repetitions on each side.

OUTER AND INNER THIGH MUSCLES

The abductors and adductors are the two muscle groups responsible for the tone on the outer and inner thighs. The abductors move the leg away from the midline of the body while the adductors pull the leg toward the midline. The great thing about these exercises is that not only do they tone the thighs, but you get a wonderful water massage at the same time – improving circulation and reducing water retention.

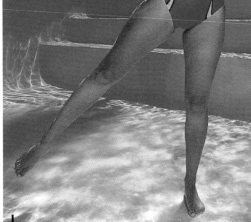

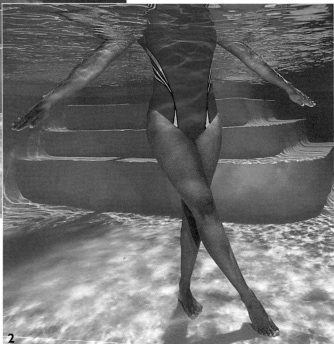

SIDE LEG RAISES AND CROSSOVERS

Start from a neutral position in chest-deep water, with the feet hip-width apart. Raise the right leg out to the side, no higher than 45° **1**. The knee faces forward. Keep the abdominals contracted and the shoulders back and down. Arms are out to the sides.

Exhaling, bring the right leg in and across, in front of the left leg **2**. (If you have had hip replacement surgery, stop at the neutral position.) Keep your arms out to the sides to stabilize. Return to neutral. You can repeat this exercise on the same side or on alternate sides. Start with two sets of eight repetitions.

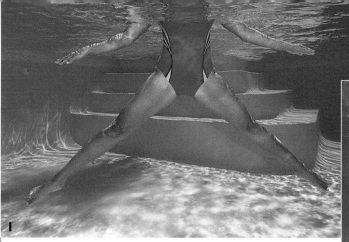

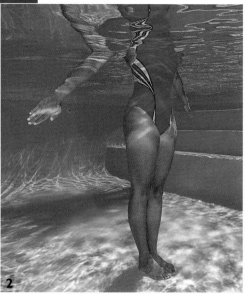

FLOATING DOUBLE LEG RAISES

Start from a neutral position, with feet together and arms out to the sides. Jump, extending both legs out to roughly 45° **1**. The legs are in line with the body, neither in front nor behind it. As you jump, keep the abdominals tight and the back extended. Hold the position.

Return to the initial position, bringing the legs together **2**. Ensure that both feet are wholly on the floor between jumps. You'll really feel this on the inner thighs. Start with two sets of eight repetitions.

OUTER THIGH CRUNCHES

Attach aquafins to the ankles, pointing from front to back. Start from a neutral position, with the feet together and arms out to the sides. Open the legs to a maximum of 45° from the midline. Keep the legs in line with the body, with the knees facing forward. Keep the abdominals tight and the back extended. Hold the position **1**.

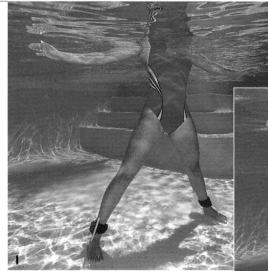

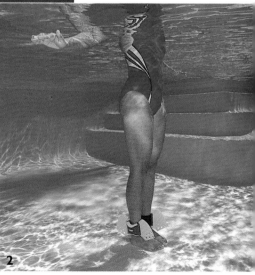

Return to the initial position, pulling in both legs **2**. Ensure that the entire foot is on the floor between jumps. Start with two sets of eight repetitions.

GLUTES AND HIP FLEXORS

The gluteus maximus (glutes) is the muscle responsible for bringing the leg back and turning it out. The glutes are everybody's bane – they can never be toned enough. The hip flexors pull the thigh forward and up. Concentrate on tightening the glutes and stretching the hip flexors: the water lets you do both at the same time.

BENT KNEE SWINGS

Starting from a neutral position, with the feet together and the arms out to the sides, raise the right knee in a front kneelift **1**. Return to neutral position **2**.

Bend the right knee and bring the foot up behind the body **3**.

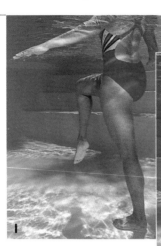
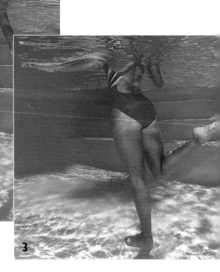
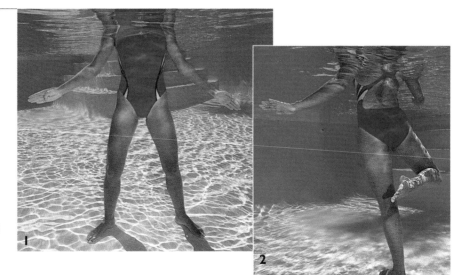

Contract the glutes by pushing the knee behind the hips. Keep the abdominals tight and do not arch the low back. Return to neutral. You can repeat this exercise on the same side or on alternate sides. Start with four sets of eight repetitions. Increase intensity by omitting Step 2.

LEG CURLS

Stand with the legs hip-width apart and the feet turned out **1**.

Turn the right leg out at the hip, bend the leg, push the knee behind the body, and the foot behind the opposite leg **2**. You can repeat on the same or on alternate sides. Start with four sets of eight repetitions.

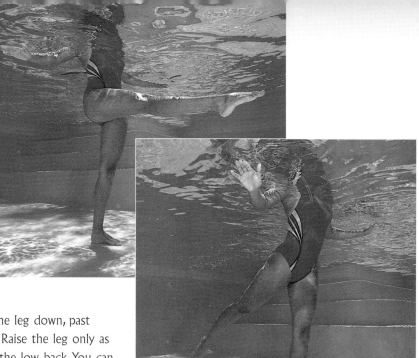

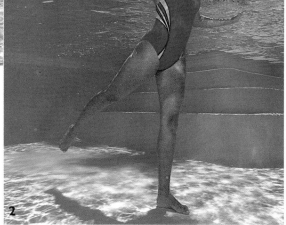

STRAIGHT LEG SWINGS

With the feet together and the arms out to the sides, raise the right leg in a front high kick. The knee faces upward. Keep the abdominals tight. Shoulders are down and back. Lift the leg only as far as you can without moving the upper body **1**.

Contracting the glutes, pull the leg down, past neutral, and into a back kick **2**. Raise the leg only as far as you can without arching the low back. You can either swing the leg forward past neutral, for another repetition, or repeat with the other leg. Start with two sets of eight repetitions per leg. (Each repetition includes one full swing to the front and the back.)

SKATES

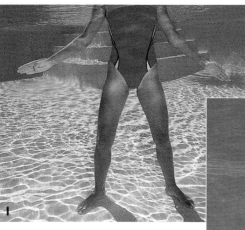

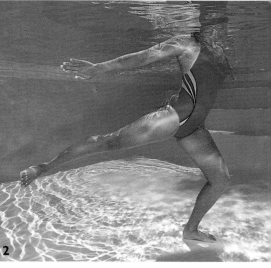

Stand with feet hip-width apart and the arms out to the sides. Keep the abdominals tight to protect the low back **1**.

Turn the right leg out at the hip, raise it, and push back as if you were skating **2**. You can push back with both arms or use complementary arms. Depending on the depth of the water, you may want to bend the support leg more or less. Raise the back leg only as far as is possible without arching the low back. Return to the start position, then repeat on the other side, turning out the left leg and pushing it back. Start with four sets of eight repetitions, alternating the leading leg. (Each repetition includes a right and a left leg raise.)

QUADS AND HAMSTRINGS

Most of your fat burning will come from these muscles. Every time you straighten out the knee, you use and quads and when you bend it, you use the hamstrings. For strong, shapely thighs, take your leg to full extension without locking the knee and bring your heel as close to the glutes as possible without arching the back.

LOW KICKS

Start from a neutral position with the feet together. Use the hands and arms to stabilize the body during the exercise. Flexing the right hip, raise the knee slightly as if about to take a step **1**.

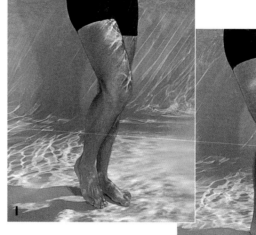
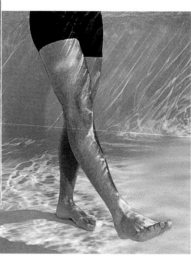

Keeping the right thigh in the same position, contract the quads to straighten the leg to the front **2**. Keep the knee joint soft. The foot can be flexed, as here, or pointed. Return to neutral position. You can repeat this exercise on the same or on alternate sides. Start with four sets of eight repetitions with each leg.

LEG CURLS

Start from a neutral position with the legs hip-width apart. Keep the abdominals tight to protect the low back. Extend the right leg to the back with only the forefoot touching the floor **1**.

Bend the right knee and raise the foot behind you, at least to knee height **2**. Keep the knee under the hip or just slightly behind it. Return the leg to neutral. You can repeat this exercise on either the same or on alternate sides. Start with four sets of eight repetitions.

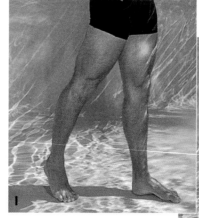

OPEN LOW KICKS

Whenever you extend the knee, you will be working all four quadriceps muscles. By turning the leg out and in, however, you can sculpt and define the outer and inner muscles of the quads. Start this exercise by turning the right hip out and raising the right knee **1**.

Keeping the right hip and thigh in the same position, straighten the leg, without locking the knee **2**. The foot can be either flexed or pointed. Return to neutral position. You can repeat this exercise on either the same or on alternate sides. Start with four sets of eight repetitions with each leg.

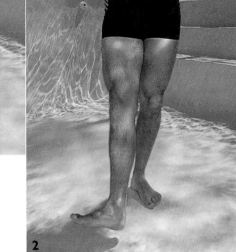

OPEN LEG CURLS (HOPSCOTCHES)

This exercise works the biceps femoris, the hamstring found on the outer side of the back of the thigh. Whenever you bend the knee, you will be working with all three hamstrings. In order to define the outer and inner hamstrings, rotate the leg out or in. Start with the feet hip-width apart, turn out the right leg, and extend it to the back **1**.

Bend the right knee and raise the foot behind you, at least to knee height **2**. Make sure that you keep the knee directly under the hip or slightly behind it. Return to neutral position. You can repeat this exercise on either the same or on alternate sides. Start with four sets of eight repetitions with each leg.

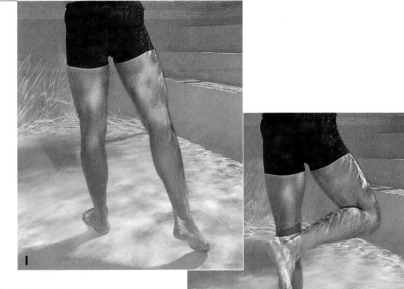

FLEXIBILITY & RELAXATION
PROGRAM

Flexibility is an important component of fitness and water is a superb medium in which to improve it. Ai Chi (created by Mr. Jun Konno of Japan, and further developed by Ms. Ruth Sova in the US) and Watsu® (created in 1980 by Mr. Harold Dull) are two aquatic disciplines that I find rewarding on many levels, including the physical, emotional, and spiritual. While it will not be possible here to teach you everything there is to know about these methods, I would like to give you at least a glimpse into this wonderful dimension of water exercise. Remember that stretching and relaxation workouts should be performed in warmer water temperatures (90–98°F / 33–37°C) to aid flexibility and joint mobility.

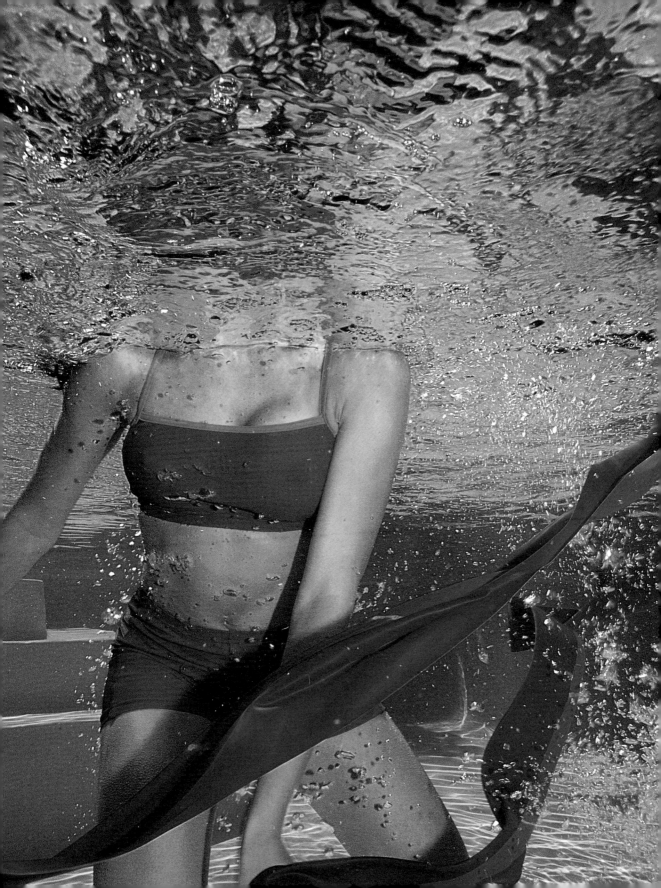

AI CHI
preparing

Ai Chi ("energy of love") is a water exercise and relaxation program that combines deep breathing and slow, large movements, performed in continuous, flowing patterns. Throughout the exercises, inhale through the nose and exhale through the nose and mouth. The three exercises here are from the first Ai Chi sequence, in which we focus on the breathing. Accompany your workout with soothing music or nature sounds.

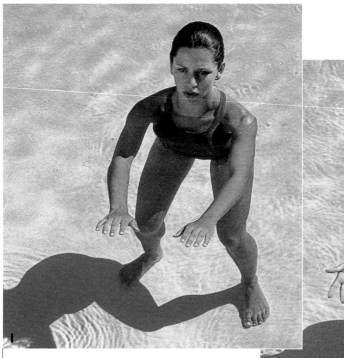

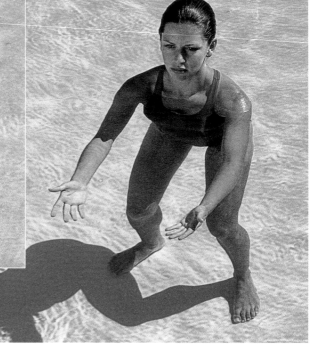

FLOATING

Allow yourself to be supported by the water's buoyancy. Inhale, then as you exhale, lower the hands with the palms down **1**.

Inhaling, raise your arms in front of you with the palms facing up **2**. Repeat 5–10 times, then exhale and lower the arms in preparation for the next movement.

In Ai Chi, each movement is a preparation for the one that follows: the exercises flow into each other with no interruptions.

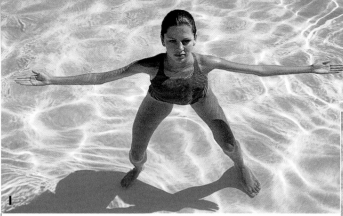

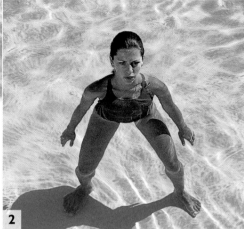

UPLIFTING

Continue from the previous exercise, with arms lowered in front of the body, palms down. Inhale and raise the arms out to the sides, bringing them to shoulder level but still under water. Palms face upward 1. The legs are in a wide stance with the knees bent and the feet slightly turned out.

Exhaling, lower the arms until they are down by your sides, palms facing inward 2. Repeat these movements 5–10 times, then lift the arms out to the sides again in preparation for the next exercise.

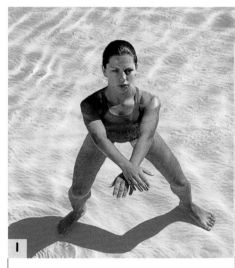

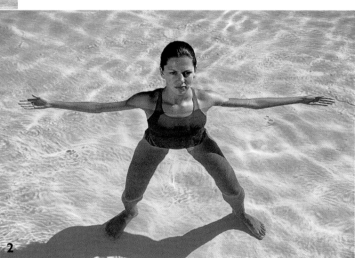

ENCLOSING

Continue from the previous exercise, with the arms out to the sides at shoulder height, palms facing up. Exhale and, turning the palms down, bring the arms in across the body at shoulder height until they cross at the wrists 1. Keep the legs in the same wide stance, with knees bent and feet slightly turned out.

Inhale and, keeping your arms at shoulder height, open them out to the sides as wide as is comfortable for you, with the palms facing upward 2. Repeat 5–10 times, then raise the arms out to the sides in preparation for the next movement (*see pp112–113*).

AI CHI
healing

The second Ai Chi sequence focuses on healing, and includes exercises for the upper and lower body and trunk stability. Repeat each movement 5–10 times, being careful to maintain correct alignment and ensuring that each movement flows into the next. Remember to inhale through the nose and exhale through the nose and mouth.

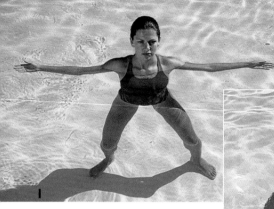

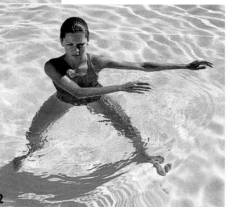

SOOTHING

Continue from the previous exercise, with the arms out to the sides at shoulder height, palms facing up **1**. As before, the legs are in a wide stance, with the knees bent and the feet slightly turned out.

Turning the palms down, exhale and bring the right arm across the chest, toward the left arm **2**.

As you inhale, turn the palms up and open the right arm to the side at shoulder height. Repeat 5–10 times, then repeat on the left. Return to initial position with arms out to the sides.

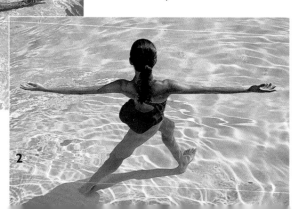

GATHERING

Exhaling, turn the palms down as you bring the right arm toward the left. Swiveling your feet around, turn the upper body to the left to face your outstretched hands **1**. Inhaling, turn the palms up and open the left arm to the back. The upper body now faces back **2**. Reverse the moves until you face left again. Repeat 5–10 times, then repeat to the right. Return to initial position, with arms out to the sides.

ACCEPTING

Exhaling, turn the palms down and, as you shift your weight onto the right leg, bring the left arm across the chest toward the right arm **1**.

Pivot both feet 90° so you are facing right. The weight is now evenly balanced on both legs **2**.

As you inhale, turn the palms upward and open both arms out to the sides at shoulder height, pulling them back and shifting your weight onto the back leg **3**. Stabilize the trunk.

Exhaling, turn the palms down and bring the arms out in front of you, again shifting the weight forward. Repeat the last two movements 5–10 times then return to center. Repeat to the left then return to the initial position with the arms out to the sides.

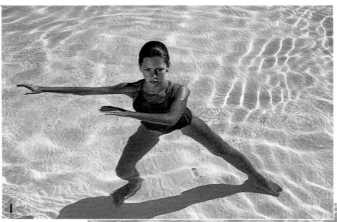

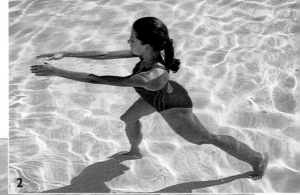

AI CHI
healing

The focus now shifts to the lower body and balance. Both Jun Konno and
Ruth Sova believe that Ai Chi should be for everyone. There is no wrong
way: the way that feels best for you is the right way. Whatever adaptations
you make to Ai Chi will make it right for you. Don't forget your breathing.

ACCEPTING WITH GRACE,

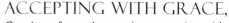

Continue from the previous exercise, with the arms
out to the sides at shoulder level, palms facing down
1. As before, the legs are in a wide stance with the
knees bent and the feet slightly turned out.

Exhaling, bring your left arm to the right so the
thumbs touch. Pivot both feet 90° so you face right.
Your weight is evenly balanced on both legs 2.

Inhale and open the arms at shoulder level, palms
up. At the same time, shift your weight back onto
the left leg and raise your right leg in front 3.

Exhaling, turn the palms down and
bring the arms forward at shoulder height
while you lower your leg. Repeat the last
two movements 5–10 times, then repeat
on the other side. Return to the initial
position with the arms out to the sides.

ROUNDING

Continuing from the previous exercise, bring the left arm to the right and turn to face right. Inhaling, turn the palms up, pull the arms back, and shift your weight to your back leg **1**.

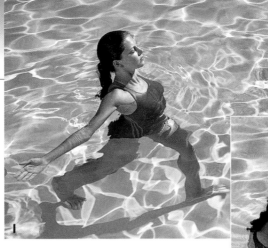

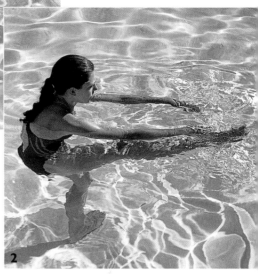

Exhaling, turn the palms down and bring your arms forward until the thumbs touch. At the same time, bring the back leg forward and raise it in front of you, trying to touch your toe with your fingertips **2**. Repeat the movement 5–10 times, then return to center. Repeat on the other side, then return to the initial position with the arms out to the sides.

BALANCING

Continuing from the previous exercise, bring the left arm to the right and turn to face right. Inhaling, turn the palms up, pressing both arms down and back. Lead with the back of the hand, palms facing forward. At the same time bring the back leg forward in a high kick and lean slightly backward **1**.

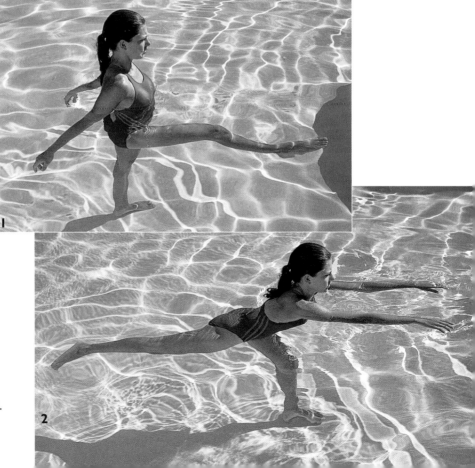

Exhaling, turn the palms down, pull the arms forward and up, and extend the right leg down and back. Lean forward **2**. Repeat these two movements 5–10 times, then repeat on the left. Return to center with arms by the sides.

AI CHI
cultivating the chi

These two exercises are from the fourth Ai Chi sequence, Cultivating the Chi, in which we hold the life energy and nurture it. If you enjoy this introductory experience of Ai Chi and would like to learn more, contact the Aquatic Therapy and Rehabilitation Institute (ATRI) (*see p157*).

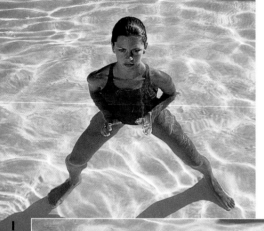

SURROUNDING

Stand in a wide stance, supported by the water as before. Hold your hands in front of you, palms facing each other, as if you were holding a ball of life energy (chi) that you have gathered in the water **1**.

Exhaling, and pivoting to the left, move your hands so the right hand moves above the "ball" and the left is below it **2**.

Keep turning until your legs cross and you are facing in the opposite direction **3**. Visualize surrounding yourself with chi. Inhale and turn in the opposite direction to come back to center and the initial position.

Exhaling, repeat the exercise, turning to the right. Repeat the exercise three times in both directions, watching your hands all the time.

The ball of "chi" is held by the left hand underneath and the right hand above.

NURTURING

Start as before, with the arms open to the sides at shoulder height, palms turned down **1**.

Bringing the right arm towards the left, pivot the feet to turn 90° to the left. As you exhale, bend the knees and lean forward. Pushing the hands and arms forward slightly, let them sink down in the water **2**.

Inhaling, straighten the knees and raise the hands in front of the body, palms up **3**. Repeat the last two movements three times.

Return to center and repeat in the opposite direction. With each breath, you will be eliminating stress and filling your reserves with clean, fresh chi.

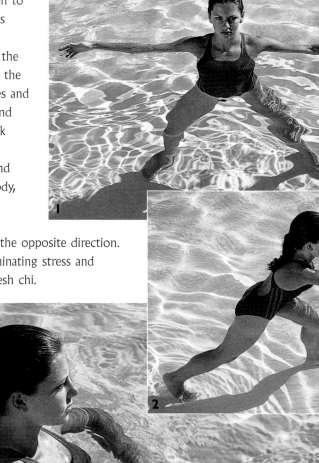

WATSU®

At its simplest level, Watsu® (Water Shiatsu) is a floating massage. However, it is the water, not the giver, that massages the receiver. Combining elements of Zen Shiatsu (a Japanese massage technique) with floating in a warm pool, Watsu® fosters serenity and bliss for both giver and receiver. I have illustrated here parts of various simple sequences. Repeat each movement 3–5 times before passing to the next movement in the sequence.

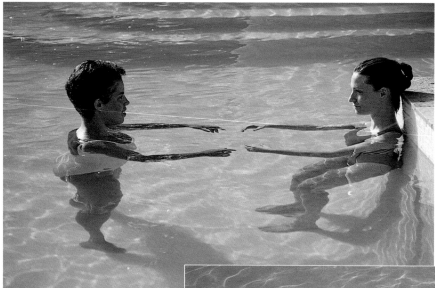

WATER BREATH DANCE AND BREATH ROCK

2 With her arm over the receiver's right shoulder and under her head, the giver positions the receiver in the water. They breathe in unison, and the giver gently rocks the receiver back and forth in the water.

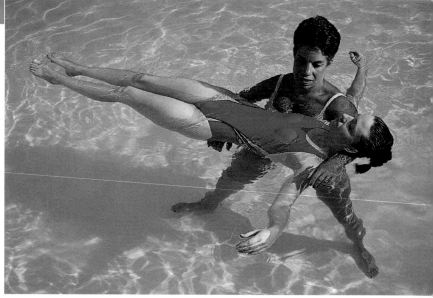

OPENING THE BASIC FLOW

1 Start the session by having the receiver lean against the pool wall as if seated. Before touching the receiver, the giver informs her that the next time she will be in this position, the session will be coming to an end. The giver encourages the receiver to relax and to concentrate on her breathing before the first sequence begins.

ACCORDION

3 With the receiver cradled in her arms, the giver opens and closes her arms, "folding" and "unfolding" the receiver. Their breathing is coordinated with the movements, inhaling as the arms open and the receiver lengthens, exhaling as the arms close and the receiver folds in.

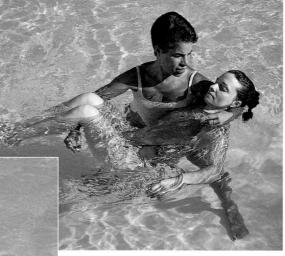

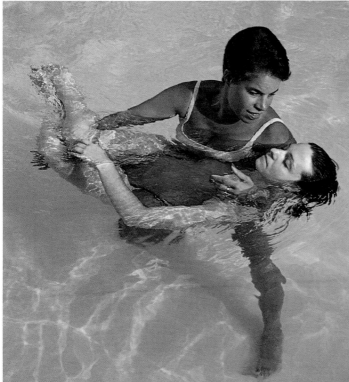

ROTATING ACCORDION

4 Once the receiver is folded, the giver pushes her legs away from her body. When the legs are at their furthest, the hips swing away from the giver, who pulls the legs back toward her body. At the same time the giver twists from side to side and continues to fold and unfold the receiver, twisting, opening, and swaying.

NEAR-LEG ROTATION

5 As the giver drops back and opens her arms, she lets the far leg slip off her arm. She continues to rotate the near leg to the opposite shoulder, folding and swaying. As she drops back and pulls the near leg toward her, the far leg is stretched by the water's resistance.

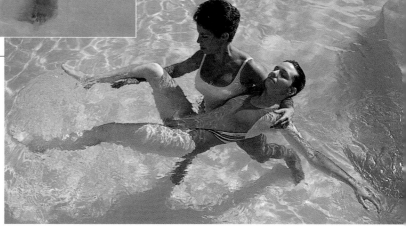

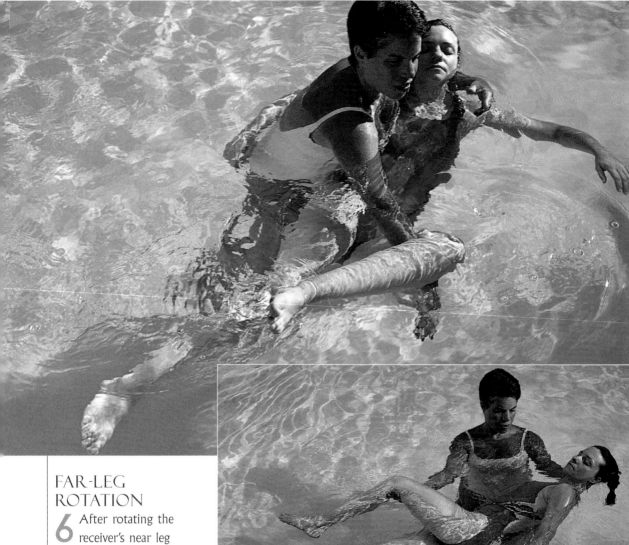

FAR-LEG ROTATION

6 After rotating the receiver's near leg (*see pp118–119*), the giver releases it and scoops up the far leg. She then repeats the same rhythmic rotation. Again, the breathing of the giver and the receiver are coordinated as the bodywork experience continues for both.

HEAD CRADLE

7 Holding the receiver under her head and under the knee of the far leg, the giver rocks the receiver in the water. (Never hold the receiver by the neck, since this is uncomfortable and potentially dangerous.)

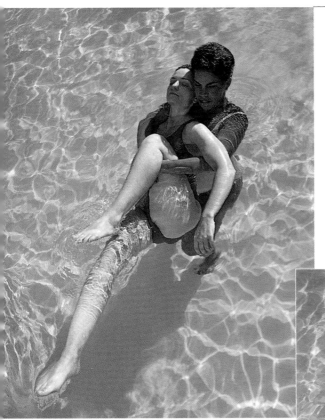

THIGH PRESS

8 Sliding the receiver's far leg onto her forearm, the giver turns her around so that her back is against her chest. Holding the thigh with both arms, the giver presses the thigh into the receiver's chest, stretching her low back, and holds for a few seconds.

SEAWEED

9 Now the giver stays as low as possible in the water. Releasing the thigh, she places the receiver's head on her shoulder, holding her hips with both hands if possible. Slowly the giver pushes the receiver's hips from side to side.

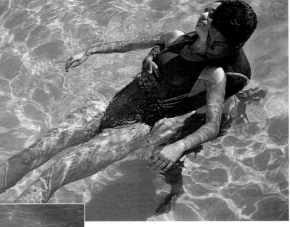

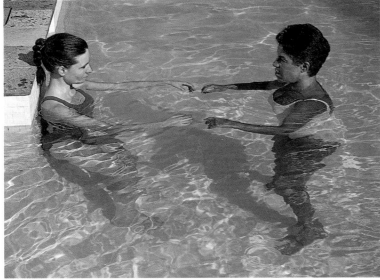

WALL RETURN

10 At the end of these sequences, the receiver is repositioned against the wall, where she can collect her bearings. Many people fall asleep during a Watsu® session, so some time is needed to return to reality. The giver faces her in the water, honoring the receiver's space, and remaining close to her, still united despite the separation.

ON THE BEACH

When the summer rolls around and you are on your hard-earned vacation, you may find the energy for a bit of exercise. The water is there and you'll also have another ally — the sand. These are the perfect ingredients for a workout. To inspire you, here are some exercises that use the resistance of the sand and the force of the waves to give you an invigorating and enjoyable workout.

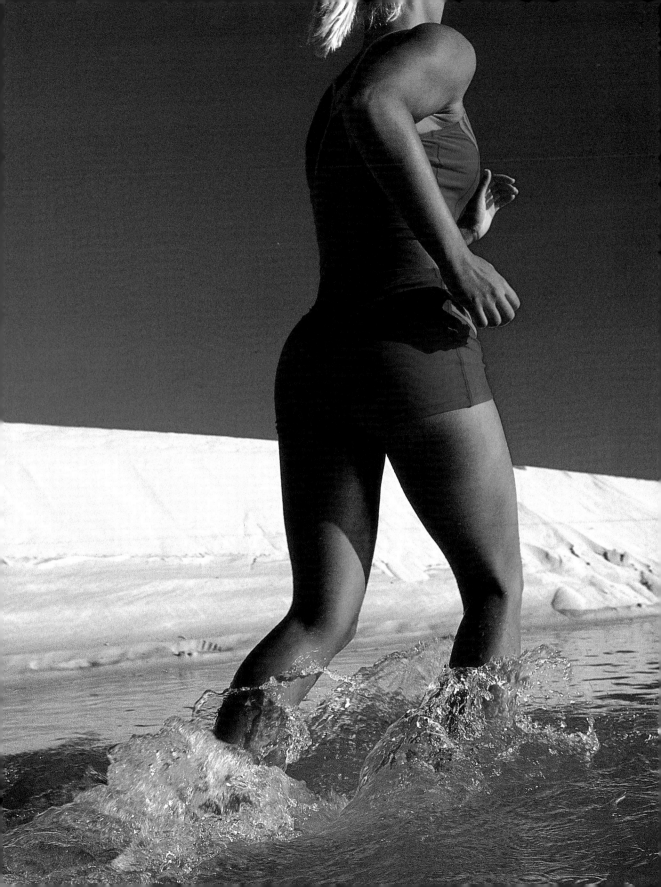

USING THE SAND

Here are some great muscle-toning exercises that you can try out on the beach, using the sand as your workload. Because of the range of movements involved in these exercises, you will also be working on your hip mobility. You can work in dry or wet sand – both will provide a great resistance for the working muscles. To increase the resistance, dig the working foot deeper into the sand.

CAUTION Keep the abdominals tight and your back in neutral alignment throughout. Keep the support leg slightly bent and maintain the correct hip-knee-foot alignment of the working leg.

INTENSITY Increase intensity by digging deeper and moving more sand with each stroke, in all directions.

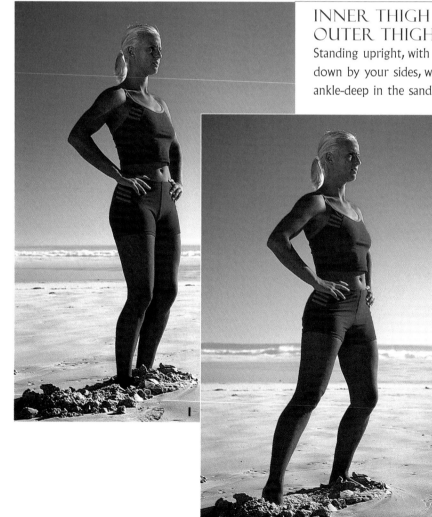

INNER THIGH CRUNCH AND OUTER THIGH PRESS

Standing upright, with your hands on your hips or down by your sides, wiggle your feet until they are ankle-deep in the sand **1**. Hold your abdominals tight and stabilize the trunk. The knees are soft.

Bend the supporting leg then, exhaling, push the sand out to the side with your right foot **2**. Keep moving the foot sideways until it stops pushing the sand. Make sure that you push the foot straight to the side.

Inhale then, exhaling, bring the leg back in toward the left leg, pushing the sand in toward the leg and burying the foot even deeper. Inhale.

Start with three sets of eight repetitions, then repeat on the other side.

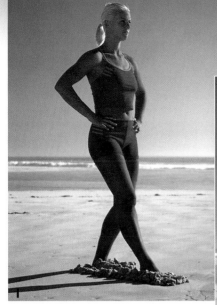

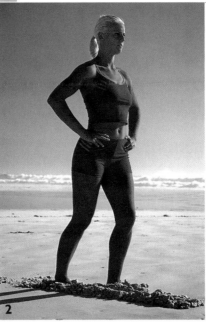

LEG EXTENSIONS/ REAR CRUNCHES

Start as before. Bend both legs. Exhaling, straighten the knee of the right leg, pushing the sand forward with the foot **1**. Do not lock the knee. Inhale.

Exhaling, dig the heel into the sand, bend the knee slightly, and pull the leg back behind you **2**. Straighten the knee and inhale. Repeat three sets of eight repetitions, then repeat on the other side.

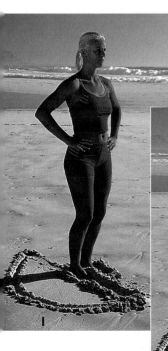

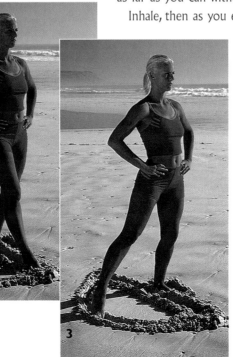

HIP MOBILITY

Standing upright with your hands on your hips, wiggle your feet until they are ankle-deep in the sand. Hips are square to the front. Bend the support leg **1**.

Exhaling, extend the right leg forward, pushing the sand with the foot. Take it as far as you can without locking the knee **2**.

Inhale, then as you exhale, move the leg around in a semicircle, pushing the sand with the foot. **3**. Keep circling the foot until it is back as far as you find comfortable. Inhale, then, exhaling again, pull the leg forward, pushing the sand.

After eight repetitions with the right leg, repeat with the left. Alternating sides, perform six sets of eight repetitions, three on each side.

AGAINST THE WAVES

The sun is shining, the sea is sparkling, and you can't resist getting into the water. Once you are in there, playing with the waves, you will get a great workout for all the trunk muscles. The waves provide the turbulence necessary to increase the intensity of these exercises and, after the wave has hit you, you will have to resist the force of the ebb and flow of the tide.

CAUTION These exercises are only for swimmers or those who have the confidence to work out in the breakers. The exercises are tiring because you will be contracting and stretching muscles continuously to maintain balance and core stability against the turbulence of the water. Don't overdo it. When you are tired, relax. Listen to your body.

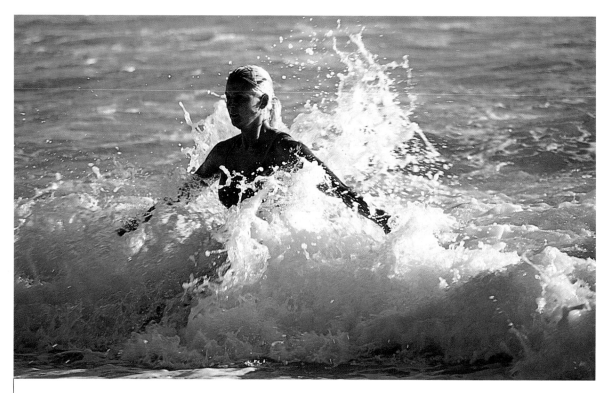

BACK TO THE WAVES

Bracing yourself against the force of the breakers and the ebb and flow of the tide provides a great opportunity for a workout. Stand with your back to the waves, where the waves are breaking. Make sure that you are at least hip-deep in the still water. Dig your feet into the sand so that you have a good stable stance. When the waves hit, extend the spine, keeping the abdominals tight. At the same time, pull back the arms, flexing and extending the elbows to condition the biceps and triceps in the turbulence of the breaking waves.

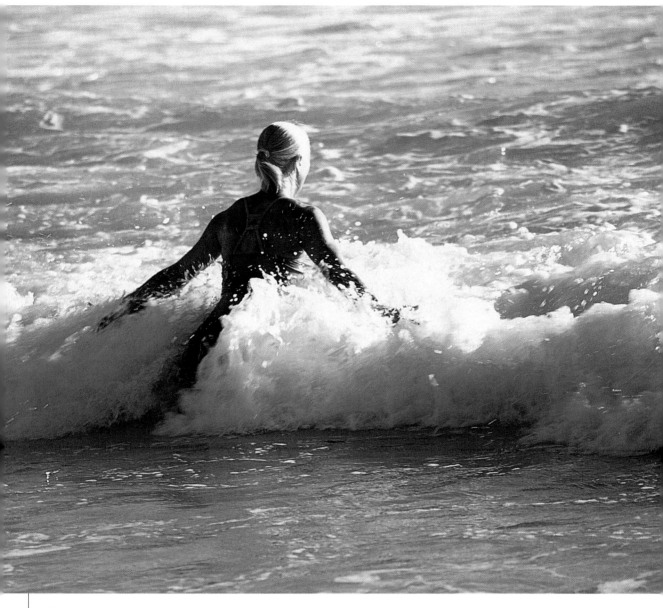

FACING THE WAVES

These movements are similar to those in the preceding exercise, but now you can prepare yourself for the force of the breakers. Position yourself so that the turbulence of the breaking waves is against your abdomen. Stand in a good stabilizing position with your feet rooted to the ground and your arms out to the sides. When the wave breaks and hits you, pull your arms in front of you, flexing and extending the arms to work the biceps, triceps, pecs, and deltoids in the turbulence of the water. Stabilize the trunk muscles and the legs.

SHALLOW-WATER EXERCISES

Exercising in even shallow water can be wonderfully beneficial – movements that are difficult on land can be done to perfection in just a little water. As you continue practicing these exercises, gradually move into shallower water, then onto land.

CAUTION Keep the abdominals contracted to protect the low back. Keep the shoulders down and the head in alignment with the spine.

INTENSITY Each time you do these exercises in shallower water, you will be working harder. If there is any current where you are exercising, this will also increase the intensity of the movements.

STRAIGHT LEG L-PRESS

Sit in water that covers your shoulders. Extend the legs so your body forms an "L" shape **1**.

Contract the quads and abdominals and, as you exhale, push off the floor, supporting your body weight with your arms **2**. Lower yourself back down, controlling the return. Repeat eight times, holding the raised position. Repeat in progressively shallower water.

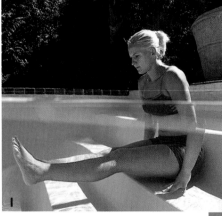

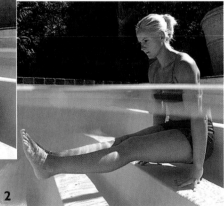

PUSH-UP

Start in a prone position in water that covers the shoulders. Hands are under the shoulders. Keep the abdominals tight and the shoulders back and down **1**.

Push up, straightening the arms. The back is in neutral alignment. **2**.

Return to the starting position. Start with one set of 12 repetitions, then move to shallower water and repeat.

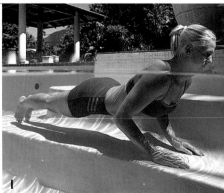

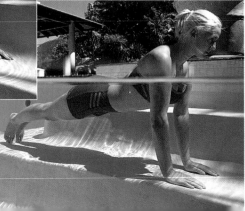

ROLLING TRICEPS PUSH-UP

Start in a prone position in water that covers your shoulders. Elbows are on the floor, under the shoulders, and the forearms are straight to the front, flat on the floor. The tips of the toes rest on the floor. Keep the abdominals contracted and your head in alignment with the spine **1**.

Keeping your elbows close to the body and hands flat on the floor, pull your body forward so that the elbows come off the ground next to the ribs and the shoulders are over the hands **2**.

Extend the arms until they are straight. Do not hyperextend or lock the elbows. Keep the shoulders down and the head in alignment with the spine. **3** Slowly bend the elbows, lowering the body back to the starting position. Repeat at least eight times, then repeat in shallower water.

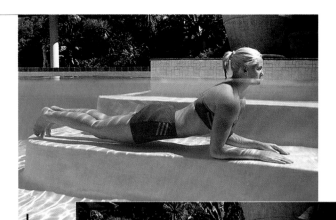

1

2

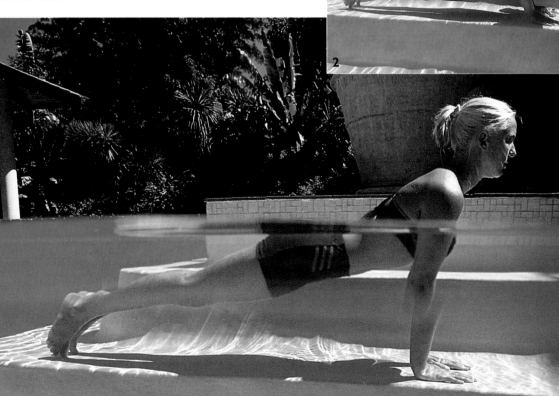

3

DEEP-WATER EXERCISES

When you are at the beach, provided you are a confident swimmer, you can easily work out in deep water, even without flotation equipment. The density of the salt water will keep you buoyant and, as long as you keep your arms and legs moving, you will stay afloat and keep warm.

CAUTION Working without a flotation belt, these exercises are for swimmers only. Keep the abdominals tight, the shoulders back and down, and the back in neutral alignment.

INTENSITY Increase intensity by wearing webbed gloves or aquafins. Another alternative is to not use the arms at all, but move only with the strength of the legs.

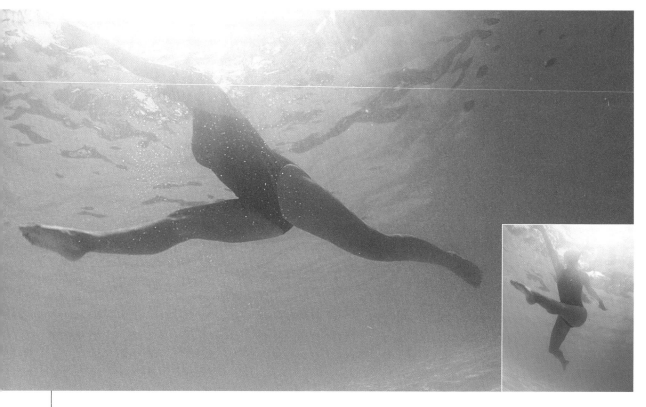

THE GAZELLE

Once you are out in deep water, bring the right knee up in a knee-lift, then extend the leg forward in a huge leap. The left leg extends back. The left arm comes forward as the right arm goes back. Pull the left leg forward to a front kneelift while the right leg pushes down against the water and back. The left leg now extends forward. Keep the upper body erect as you travel forward in the water.

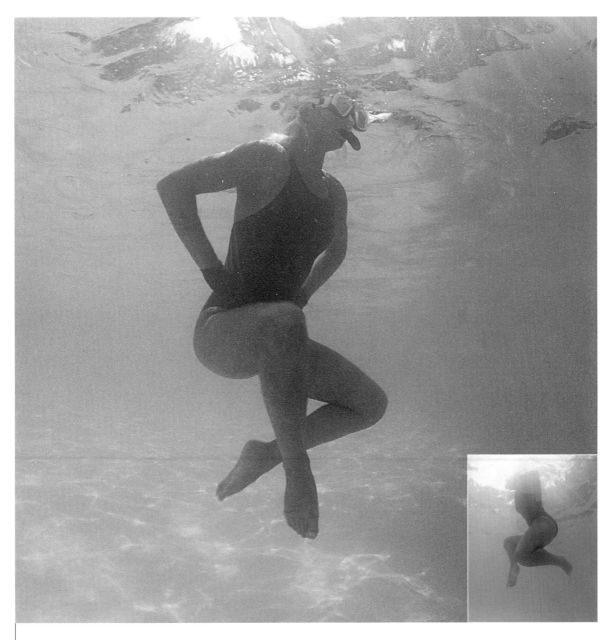

THE 360°

This exercise will have you turning in circles, through 360°. Once you're in deep water, turn the right hip out and the left hip in, bend the knees, and bring them up. The right knee will be in front of you and the left will be slightly behind you. Repeatedly extend and bend the knees to kick yourself in a circle. Once you have turned full circle, turn the legs in the opposite direction (left hip out and right hip in) and kick yourself in a circle in the opposite direction.

SPORT-SPECIFIC EXERCISES

Are you preparing to participate in some special sporting event? As well as your regular training program, you will find cross-training in the water particularly beneficial. By performing sport-specific moves against the resistance and buoyancy of the water, you will train both your muscles and your nervous system to perform better and react faster. Even if you're not in training, and sport is just an occasional pastime, you will still find these exercises great fun.

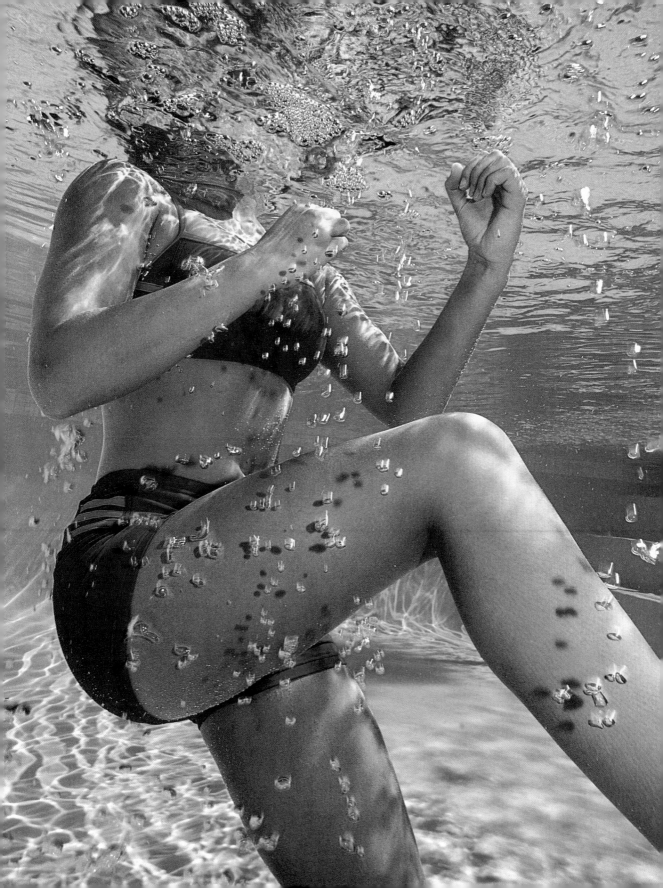

SWIMMING

Just as a change from swimming in your usual horizontal position in water, try some vertical exercises to enhance your performance. Standing upright in shoulder-depth water, or suspended vertically in deep water, you can practice the crawl, the backstroke, and the butterfly. Without putting any strain on the shoulder joint, you can exercise and strengthen the muscles involved in these popular swimming strokes.

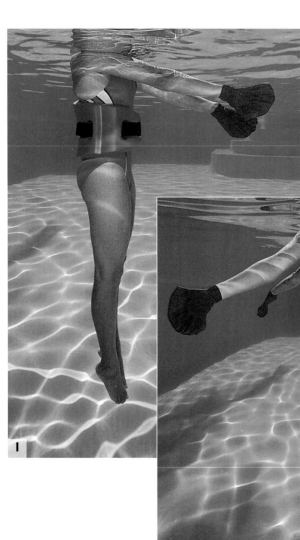

CRAWL

Work in deep water, wearing a flotation belt and webbed gloves or aquafins on your wrists. Maintain a vertical position in the water, with the feet pointing straight down to the pool floor. Begin the exercise by bringing both arms forward, leading with the back of the hand **1**.

Pull your arms straight back, leading with the palm of the hand **2**. When you reach the maximum extension, rotate the arm so the palm faces downward and pull the arm forward, back to the starting position. Repeat the movement and you will find that you are traveling forward. Start by doing two pool lengths and increase gradually. In this exercise, the arms can work bilaterally, as shown here, or unilaterally, to mimic the crawl.

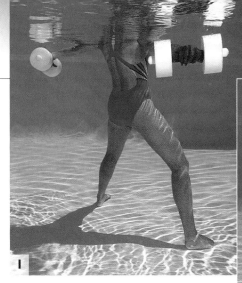

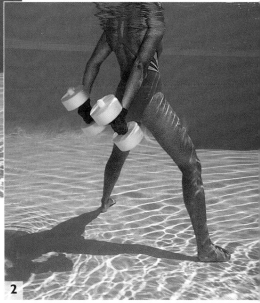

BACKSTROKE

Work in chest-depth water, holding a hand-bar in each hand. If you want to further increase the intensity, you can also wear webbed gloves.

Stand in the stabilizing position of your choice, with your arms out to the sides at shoulder level **1**. Keep your abdominals very tight, your legs bent, and your feet rooted to the ground.

Exhaling, pull the arms down and back until the hands meet at the back **2**. Hold this position for 2 seconds, then release and slowly bring the arms back to the original position.

BUTTERFLY

Work in shoulder-depth water, wearing webbed gloves. Start in the lunge stabilizing position (*see p23*), with the arms up in front of the body at shoulder height **1**. Tighten the abdominals and root your feet to the floor.

Exhaling, begin to pull your arms down. Keep the abdominals tight as you pull. Keep the shoulders down and back and the head in alignment with the spine **2**.

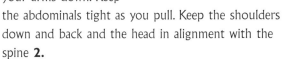

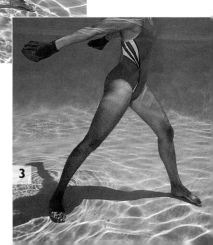

Continue bringing the arms down and back as far as is comfortable for you. Once they reach the fully extended position, turn them so the hands are palms down **3**. Inhaling, pull the arms forward and out of the water (as in the butterfly stroke) just above the water's surface, and reposition them gently on the water's surface.

WALKING, JOGGING, STRIDING, CYCLING

These aerobic exercises will tone your heart and burn lots of calories but, unlike high-impact work on land, they will cause no strain on the knees, hips, and back. After a workout against the resistance of water, you'll feel as if you are flying once you're back on land. The deeper the water, the harder you have to work to move through it.

WALKING

Wearing aquafins to increase intensity, walk normally in chest- to shoulder-depth water. Maintain erect posture and swing your arms 1.

As you get stronger, take larger strides and walk in deeper water 2. The challenge then is to keep your feet on the ground and maintain an erect posture. Start by walking lengths of the pool for 10 minutes, then increase until you are walking for 20 minutes.

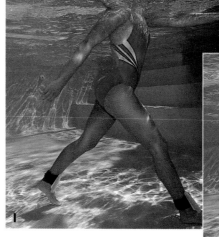
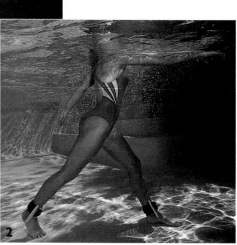

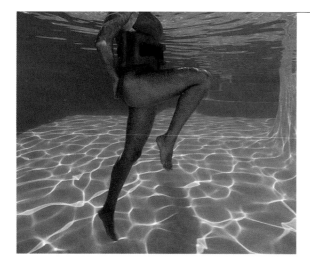

DEEP-WATER JOG

Wearing a flotation belt, start to jog, raising the right knee to hip height and pushing down and back with the left leg. The tendency in this exercise is to go horizontal: try to maintain an erect posture and neutral alignment. Hold your abdominals tight, keep your shoulders back and down, and lead with the chest. Pump the arms as if you were running on land. You can cup the hands to increase the intensity on the arms and upper body.

Start by jogging the length of the pool eight times; then increase until you can jog nonstop for 20 minutes.

DEEP-WATER STRIDING

This exercise is for swimmers who are confident in
deep water without a flotation belt. With your arms
extended, hold a woggle — either in front of the
body or behind, as here. Stay upright and take large
strides, extending one leg to the front as the other
pushes back through the water, into what seems like
a split. Start by striding the length of the pool eight
times, then increase until you can stride nonstop for
20 minutes.

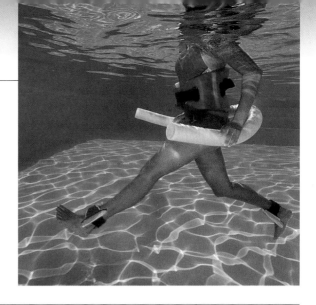

DEEP-WATER CYCLING

For this exercise, you will again be in deep water,
wearing a flotation belt. Maintaining an upright
posture, hold your hands behind your back. Keep
your shoulders back and down, your elbows back,
and your head in alignment with the spine. Start
pedaling. The legs will be working in opposition but
both legs push forward, down, and back as the knees
bend and straighten. Pedal at a brisk pace. As you
pedal, you will move forward. Start by cycling the
length of the pool eight times, then increase until
you can cycle nonstop for 20 minutes.

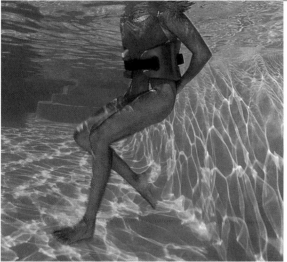

DEEP-WATER CYCLING
WITH WOGGLE

Again, this exercise is for those who feel comfortable
in deep water without a flotation belt. Keeping the
arms extended, hold on to a woggle behind you. Do
not lock the elbows. Keep the shoulders down and
back and the head in alignment with the spine. Start
cycling, as in the exercise above: besides keeping you
afloat, the woggle is the load that you have to pull
behind you as you move forward. Start by cycling
the length of the pool eight times, then increase
until you can cycle nonstop for 20 minutes.

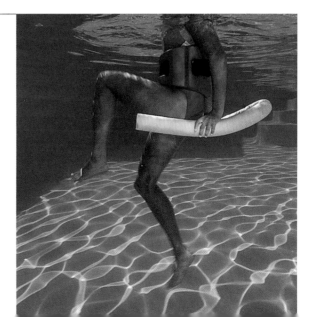

SKIING, SNOWBOARDING

You may wonder how you can do a pre-ski workout in water – there aren't any pools that go downhill! That's an old joke, but in fact you can prepare very well for the ski season in the pool. Skiing is a skill that mainly involves balance, and we can certainly train for balance in the pool using buoyancy equipment for flotation. All these exercises are for swimmers who feel confident in deep water without a flotation belt.

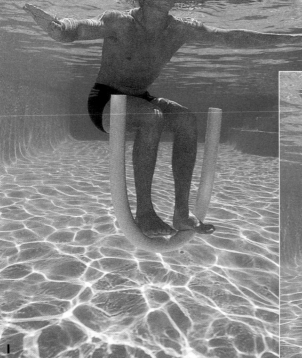

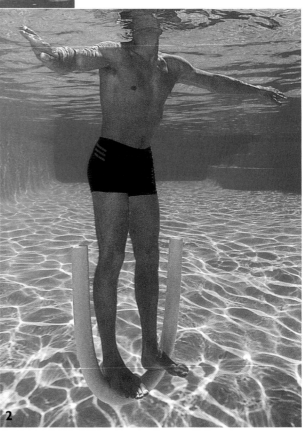

DEEP-WATER SQUAT

In deep water, stand on a woggle with your feet hip-width apart and your arms out to the sides in a stabilizing position. Maintain the woggle directly under your body. Controlling the upward thrust of the woggle, bend your legs into a squat **1**. Push the woggle down toward the floor. Stay erect, contracting the abdominals, glutes, and quads. If you feel you are losing your balance at any time, pull your legs up under your body, stabilize, and then return to the starting position with legs straight **2**. Start by performing four sets of eight repetitions.

DEEP-WATER SLALOMS

Stand on the handles of a kickroller with the feet close to the roller. Arms are out to the sides, but you will use your hands to push forward in the water. Push one leg down toward the floor. Both legs are bent **1**.

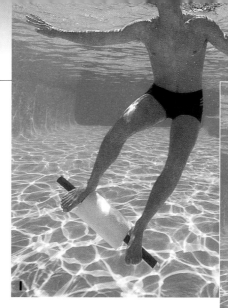

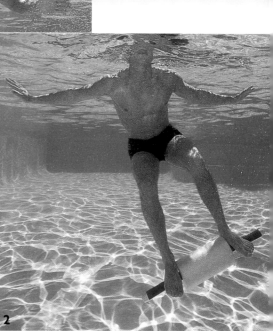

As you move forward in the water, return to center and repeat the movement on the other side **2**. As you move forward it will seem as though you are slaloming. Try slaloming the length of the pool as far as you can. If you can manage two lengths, you're doing fine.

SNOW-BOARDING

For this exercise, we use a swimbar. Keeping your feet parallel, find your balance on the swimbar and face the side of the pool. Turn your upper body so that it faces forward as your lower body continues to face the side **1**. The arms are out to the sides and will push the water back. The hips and knees are bent.

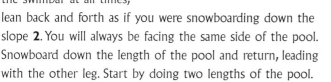

Keeping your feet on the swimbar at all times, lean back and forth as if you were snowboarding down the slope **2**. You will always be facing the same side of the pool. Snowboard down the length of the pool and return, leading with the other leg. Start by doing two lengths of the pool.

KICKBOXING

Kickboxing is now recognized as a beneficial addition to a fitness program, so let's include some of the moves in our water-based routine. Obviously, we are not preparing to do full contact, but with the right music and attitude, this martial art form can be adapted to provide a valid variation to any aquafitness program. Here are some punches and kicks that you might like to try.

JAB

Standing in shoulder-depth water, turn both feet slightly to the right; shift the shoulders so they are square with the hips and you are facing right. Bend your elbows and lift your hands in a loose fist **1**. This is ready position.

Shift the weight onto the right leg and extend the right arm in a controlled straight punch **2**. Return the arm to ready position. Perform eight complete repetitions (eight right jabs, eight left jabs).

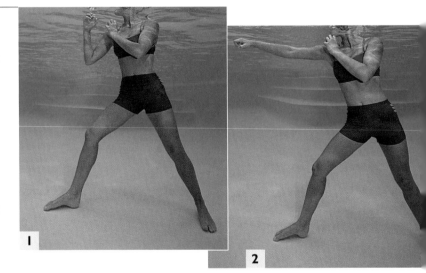

CROSS

Start in the same position as above, with the elbows bent and the hands up in a loose fist **1**. Pivot the rear foot — the movement will continue through the knee, the hip, and the back. When it reaches the shoulder, twist and lean forward, extending the right arm to the front at shoulder level **2**.

Perform eight repetitions of the right cross, then eight of the left cross. Then combine repetitions of right jab, left cross, and vice versa.

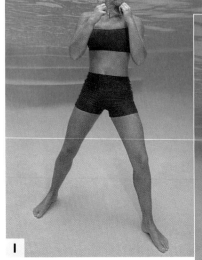

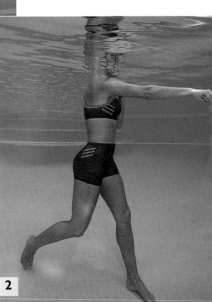

HOOK

Start as in the Cross **1**. Pivot the right foot slightly and when the movement reaches the shoulder, bring the right elbow out to the side. Keeping the arm flexed, at a right angle, bring the arm across, horizontally, until it reaches a point in front of the body's midline **2**. Return the right arm to the ready position.

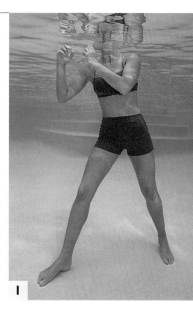

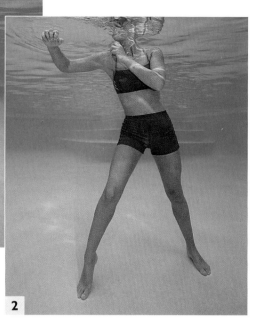

Perform eight repetitions of the right hook and eight of the left hook. Then combine repetitions of right jab, left cross, and two right hooks. Repeat on the other side.

SIDE KICK

Start with elbows bent and hands up in a loose fist. Raise the right leg in a front kneelift **1**.

Push the heel of the right foot to the side, turning the hip slightly forward until the leg is straight. Flex the knee to return to the kneelift position, and lower the leg to the floor **2**. Repeat on the other side.

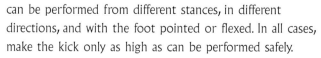

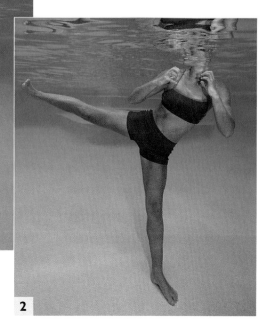

All kicks start with a front kneelift, but they can be performed from different stances, in different directions, and with the foot pointed or flexed. In all cases, make the kick only as high as can be performed safely.

GOLF, TENNIS

Golfers and tennis players have long known about the benefits to be gained from cross-training in the pool. Indeed, they even bring their rackets and clubs with them to make the training more realistic. For all these exercises, the depth of water in which you choose to work depends on your ability to control your movements. However, chest-depth is best for a good workout. Keep your arms and hands under the water.

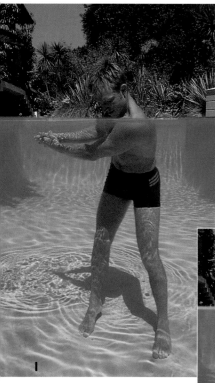

GOLF SWING

Stand in chest-deep water with the feet hip-width apart and the knees soft. Tighten the abdominals and pull back the arms to initiate the swing **1**. Do not take your arms out of the water, because the difference in the resistance can cause injury to the shoulder joint.

Keeping the hands together, palm to palm, start to strike the imaginary ball on the pool floor **2**. The open, unclenched hands will increase the resistance of the swing.

Follow the move through, shifting the weight and twisting the upper body **3**. To maintain muscle balance, try repeating the exercise in the opposite direction. Start with eight repetitions on each side.

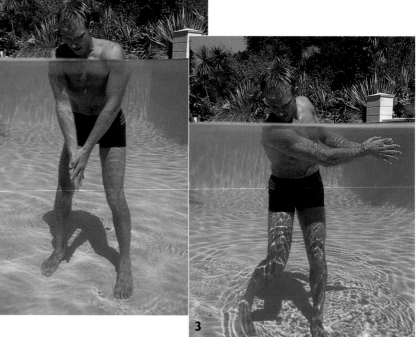

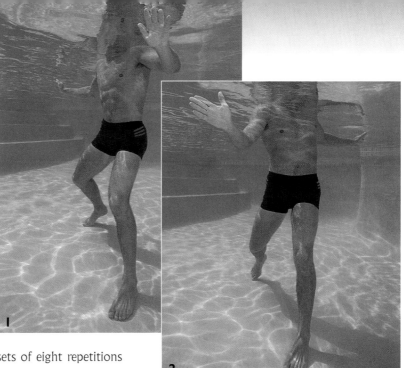

TENNIS FOREHAND

Stand in chest-deep water with the feet hip-width apart and the knees soft. Step back with the dominant leg (here the right), shifting the weight back, and bring the dominant arm (here the right) to the back, at shoulder level **1**.

Shifting the weight forward, pull the arm forward as if you had a racket in your hand **2**. Complete the move by following through, just as you would do on land. Start with two sets of eight repetitions per side, alternating sides.

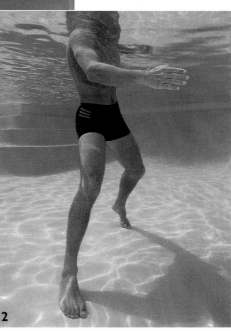

TENNIS BACKHAND

Stand in chest-deep water with the feet hip-width apart and the knees soft. Step forward with the dominant leg (here the right), pulling the dominant arm (here the right) across the body in front of the chest. Maintaining trunk stability by contracting the abdominal muscles, twist the upper body toward the back leg. Keep the hand open to increase the drag resistance **1**.

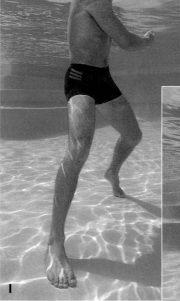

Moving forward in the water, rotate the trunk to bring it back to center. Take the arm out to the side, leading the movement with the back of the hand **2**. Continue to follow through as you would on land. As before, keep the arms under the water. Start with two sets of eight repetitions, alternating sides.

AQUA FITNESS

PROGRAMS

In the preceeding chapters, we've discussed the characteristics of water and the components of fitness; we've described the different moves that can be performed in water and ways of intensifying them; and we've learned about the various muscle groups and the exercises that target them specifically. Now we can get down to the fun of creating an exercise program that will fit your particular objectives and existing level of fitness.

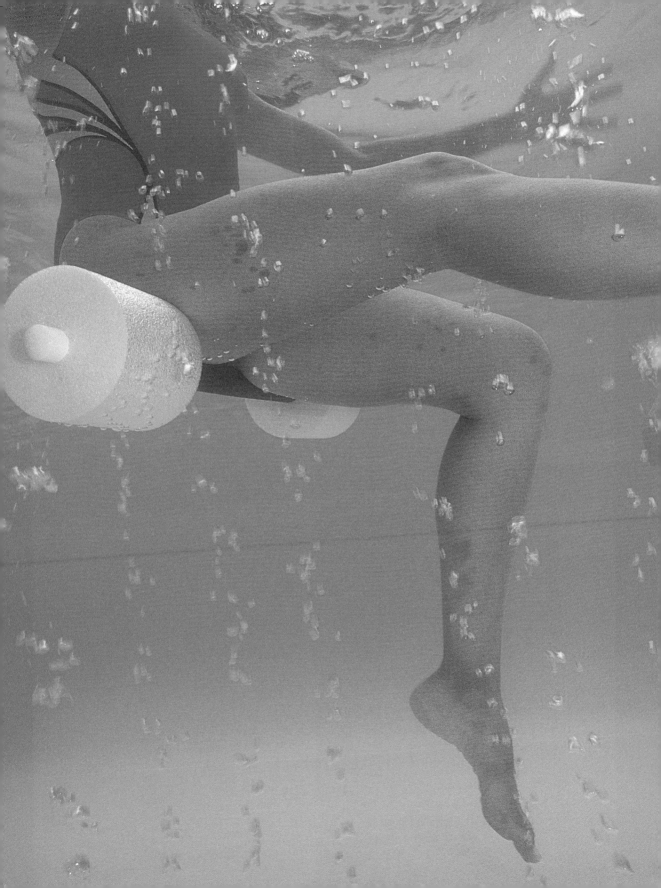

CHOOSING A PROGRAM

In water, as on land, you must follow a structured exercise program if you are to to work efficiently and progressively to enhance your fitness level. On the following pages, you will find eight different programs from which to choose. Each has a different objective, but all aim to improve your well-being safely and effectively. Try them all, and once you are familiar with how they work, try constructing your own.

To help you determine which program to try first, think about what you want from a fitness regimen: is it muscle conditioning or fat burning? Are you already quite fit and looking for a high-intensity workout? Or is this a new pursuit, which you would prefer to start slowly and work up gradually? Look through the programs and choose one that suits you and your particular requirements.

Whichever program you choose, you need to understand how the workout is structured, which muscles are being used, the principles of exercise, the use of music, and how to put it all together. All these areas have been covered in the Introduction (see pp8–33), and you may like to refer back to the relevant sections before you begin your workout. Remember that every workout starts with a warmup and ends with a cooldown.

ADD-ON CHOREOGRAPHY

If you are eager to make up your own workouts, you'll need to know more about workout choreography. If you are not, and you just want to get started on the exercises, skip the rest of this page, turn to the programs, and have fun!

Choreography can be as easy or as complex as you want it to be. Many people need music to motivate them; others just want the workout. In either case you need to know how to put the moves together logically. There are many methods, but in this book I use the most popular, basic, add-on method, which allows you to train your body in a balanced, symmetrical way.

Movement sequences are constructed by repeating the first four movements on one side, then on the other until the movements become automatic. Then another four movements are presented and repeated on both sides until they have been fully assimilated. These are added on to the first four movements and that entire sequence, or combination, is then performed. Further groups of four movements are added, and eventually the entire sequence is repeated from beginning to end. This technique is used in all the shallow- and deep-water combinations described in the book.

SYMMETRY OF MOVEMENT

Another important consideration in choreography is to ensure that both sides of the body are worked equally, so sequences are performed first with one leg, then repeated with the opposite leg. For this to work smoothly, we must prepare the lead leg. A common way of doing this is to perform two jogs and a big kick, or jog to front kick, which results in the supporting leg then being ready to go into action. The sequence goes like this:

Jog right leg up (1–2); Jog left leg up (3–4); Kick right leg to the front (5–6–7–8).
The left leg is now ready to lead the next combination with a Jog left leg up (1–2); Jog right leg up (3-4); Kick left leg to the front (5–6–7–8).

By preparing the lead leg in this way at the end of each combination you will be able to use the add-on method and plan a symmetrically balanced workout.

AEROBIC DANCE EXERCISE PROGRAM
50-MINUTE WORKOUT

At the beginning of the workout, remain stationary as you perform the movements. Once they are assimilated, you may travel back and forth or from side to side. In order to maintain aerobic intensity and continuity, flow from one movement to the next without stopping, using the arms to assist movement and increase intensity. You can alternate working at water- and half-water tempo or, sometimes, even at land tempo (see p25). If you have access to music, find tunes with speeds not exceeding 130–135 beats per minute.

Exercise	Mins	Objective	Muscle Groups	Intensity	Page
Warmup	8–10	Preparatory	All	Rhythmic limbering & static stretching	
Jog to Front Kick (Big Kick)	4	Aerobic	Hamstrings, glutes, iliopsoas, quads	Moderate	41; 42
Pendulums to Jumping Jacks	4	Aerobic	Hip abductors, adductors	Moderate	45; 47
Strides	4	Aerobic	Iliopsoas, glutes	Moderate to high	46
Open Kneelifts	4	Aerobic	Quads, sartorius	Moderate to high	40
Back Lunges	4	Aerobic	Glutes	High	46
Crossover Knee-lifts to Kicks	4	Aerobic	Obliques, adductors, quads	Moderate to high	41
Twists (arms under water)	4	Aerobic	Obliques	Moderate	48
Hopscotches to Kicks	4	Aerobic	Iliopsoas, glutes	High	43
Cool down	5	Flexibility & relaxation	All	Low	

AQUAEROBIC COMBINATION WORKOUT
50-MINUTE WORKOUT

This is a typical aquaerobic workout, similar to the one I teach. Using exercises from the Shallow-water Combinations chapter (*see pp50–69*), it provides a safe and effective aquafitness workout. As before, warm up with movements from Star 1, 2, and 3, and the appropriate stretches. Once you have completed the combination, repeat it several times, alternating the lead leg. As you work, remember to maintain your alignment, use your arms, hold in your abdominals, and try to make the movements bigger. Each time you repeat a movement, you will do it better and increase your aerobic capacity and muscular resistance.

Exercise	Mins	Objective	Muscle Groups	Intensity	Page
Warmup	8–10	Preparatory	All	Rhythmic limbering & static stretching	
Star 1	5	Aerobic	Quads, iliopsoas, hamstrings	Moderate	52
Star 2	5	Aerobic	Glutes, quads, hamstrings	Moderate	54
Star 3	5	Aerobic	Hamstrings, glutes, quads	Moderate to high	56
Star 4	5	Aerobic	Iliopsoas, sartorius, quads	Moderate to high	58
Star 5	5	Aerobic	Glutes, hamstrings, quads	High	60
Star 6	5	Aerobic	Obliques, adductors, quads	High	62
Superstar	5	Aerobic	Entire thigh	High	64
Cooldown	5	Flexibility & relaxation	All	Low	

AEROBIC DANCE AND MUSCLE-CONDITIONING WORKOUT 60-MINUTE WORKOUT

Start with an 8-minute warmup of rhythmic limbering exercises, including movements from Star 1, Star 2 and Star 3, as well as low back, lat, quad, hamstring and calf stretches. Initiate each repetition of the combination with alternate legs. If you want to work to music, choose something at about 130 beats per minute, and try to work on the beat. Remember that the bigger the movement, the more intense the exercise will be.

Exercise	Mins	Objective	Muscle Groups	Intensity	Page
Warmup	8	Preparatory	All	Rhythmic limbering & static stretching	
Star 1	2	Aerobic	Quads, iliopsoas, hamstrings	Low to moderate	52
Star 2	2	Aerobic	Glutes, quads, hamstrings	Moderate	54
Star 1 & 2	3	Aerobic		Moderate	
Star 3	2	Aerobic	Hamstrings, glutes, quads	Moderate	56
Star 1, 2 & 3	3	Aerobic		Moderate	
Star 4	2	Aerobic	Iliopsoas, sartorius, quads	Moderate	58
Star 1, 2, 3 & 4	3	Aerobic		Moderately intense	
Star 5	2	Aerobic	Glutes, quads, hamstrings	Moderately intense	60
Star 1, 2, 3, 4 & 5	4	Aerobic		High	
Star 6	2	Aerobic	Obliques, quads, adductors	High	62
Star 1, 2, 3, 4, 5 & 6	4	Aerobic		High	
Jumping Jack Combination	2	Aerobic	Abductors, adductors	High	66
Star 1, 2, 3, 4, 5, 6 & J/Jack Combination	6	Aerobic		High	
Bilateral Cross-overs & Pullbacks	3	Muscle-conditioning	Pecs, traps, rhomboid	Moderately intense	94
Shoulder Front Raises/Pressback & Lateral Raises & Pulldowns	3	Muscle-conditioning	Lats, delts	Moderately intense	96
Standing Crunch & Upper Body Twist	4	Muscle-conditioning	Abs	Moderately intense	98; 100
Cooldown	5	Flexibility & relaxation	All		

AEROBIC CIRCUIT TRAINING PROGRAM
55-MINUTE WORKOUT (3:1.5 AEROBIC: MUSCLE-CONDITIONING)

Start with a warmup of rhythmic, limbering exercises including Star 1, Star 2, and Star 3 plus low back stretches, lat stretches, quad, hamstring, and calf stretches. Add intensity to the workout by wearing webbed gloves and aquafins. Aquafins should fit snugly on the ankles, but be loose enough to alter the direction of the fins as necessary. When working the lower body, keep the upper body still, or at most use complementary arms so that you can move the legs more energetically. When using the upper body, hold the legs in the stabilizing position to control the core and allow a greater upper body range of motion.

Exercise	Mins	Objective	Muscle Groups	Intensity	Page
Warmup	8–10	Preparatory	All	Rhythmic limbering & static stretching	
Star 1	3	Aerobic	Quads, hamstrings	High	52
Bilateral Crossovers	1.5	Muscle-conditioning	Pecs, anterior delts	Moderate	94
Pendulum/Jumping Jacks	3	Aerobic	Abductors, adductors	High	66
Bilateral Pullbacks	1.5	Muscle-conditioning	Traps, posterior delts	Moderate	94
Star 3	3	Aerobic	Hamstrings, glutes	High	56
Lateral Raises	1.5	Muscle-conditioning	Medial delts	Moderate	96
Star 4	3	Aerobic	Quads	High	58
Lateral Pulldowns	1.5	Muscle-conditioning	Lats	Moderate	96
Star 5	3	Aerobic	Hamstrings	High	60
Shoulder Front Raises	1.5	Muscle-conditioning	Anterior delts	Moderate	96
Star 6	3	Aerobic	Quads	High	58
Shoulder Pressbacks	1.5	Muscle-conditioning	Lats	Moderate	96
Superstar	23	Aerobic	Quads, abductors, gluts, hamstrings	High	64
Triceps Kickbacks & Biceps Curls	1.5	Muscle-conditioning	Triceps, biceps	Moderate	92
Nefertiti	3	Aerobic	Hip flexors, glutes	High	68
Standing Ab Crunches	1.5	Muscle-conditioning	Rectus abdominus	Moderate	98
Cooldown/Ai Chi	5	Stretching & relaxation	All	Low	110

INTERVAL TRAINING PROGRAM
30, 45, OR 60-MINUTE WORKOUT (2:1 AEROBIC: ANAEROBIC)

This workout can be performed by the very fit at a high intensity level, with anaerobic phases and high intensity aerobic recovery. If you are new to exercise, work at high intensity aerobic phases with lower intensity aerobic recovery. The program consists of five 3-minute cycles. Repeat these, gradually increasing the intensity on the high intensity phase. Once you can perform the sequence twice, try it a third time — but monitor your exertion level and do not attempt a third sequence if, at any time, you feel that it is too strenuous. Pay special attention to your posture during both the aerobic and the anaerobic cycles. Never sacrifice posture for intensity. Cool down with Ai Chi.

Exercise	Mins	Objective	Muscle Groups	Intensity	Page
Warmup	8–10	Preparatory	All	Low	
1st Cycle					
Star 1	2	Aerobic	Quads, hamstrings	Moderate	52
Stride	1	Anaerobic	Glutes, iliopsoas	Very high	46
2nd Cycle					
Star 2	2	Aerobic	Quads, hamstrings	Moderate	54
Jumping Jacks	1	Anaerobic	Abductors, adductors	Very high	44
3rd Cycle					
Star 3	2	Aerobic	Glutes, iliopsoas	Moderate	56
Back Kicks & Skates	1	Anaerobic	Glutes, iliopsoas	Very high	40
4th Cycle					
Star 6	2	Aerobic	Adductors, iliopsoas, glutes	Moderate	62
Crossover High Kicks	1	Anaerobic	Adductors, iliopsoas, glutes	Very high	40
5th Cycle					
Star 5	2	Aerobic	Glutes, hamstrings, quads	Moderate	60
Hopscotch	1	Anaerobic	Glutes, hamstrings, quads	Very high	42
Cooldown	5	Relaxation		Low	

MUSCLE-CONDITIONING, WITH BUOYANCY EQUIPMENT 50–60-MINUTE WORKOUT

For this muscle-conditioning workout for the upper body, we use buoyancy equipment, such as woggles, handbars, swimbars, or kickrollers. When you work, push the equipment vertically down toward the pool floor and control its return to the surface. Keep the abdominals tight, the shoulders back and down, and keep the lower body moving to prevent loss of body heat. As before, we use the add-on method. Following an 8–10 minute warmup, start with the first move then add the second, and repeat both. Learn the third movement properly then add it to the first and second. Continue like this until you have exercised for 30–40 minutes. Cool down with lots of upper body stretches.

Lower Body Move	Upper Body Move	Objective	Muscle Groups	Page
Warmup	Warmup	Preparatory	All	
Jog	Push down	Aerobic & muscle-conditioning	Triceps	42
Jog to Kick	Push forward/Pull back	Aerobic & muscle-conditioning	Pecs, traps	40
Kneelift to Kick	Pull back, one arm at a time	Aerobic & muscle-conditioning	Lats, pecs, delts	40
Jumping Jacks to Air Jacks	Push down	Aerobic & muscle-conditioning	Triceps	44
Float prone in water	Push down	Muscle-conditioning	Pecs	94
Jog	Arms behind body; push down	Aerobic & muscle-conditioning	Triceps, lats	42
Pedal length of pool & back without touching bottom	Hold equipment behind body to float	Aerobic	Quads, hamstrings	137
Stabilizing position	Hold equipment in one hand; push up and down	Muscle-conditioning	Triceps	92
Stabilizing	Hold equipment in one hand in front of quad; flex spine	Muscle-conditioning	Obliques	99
Stabilizing	Hold equipment against chest; bend forward	Muscle-conditioning	Rectus abdominus	98
Cooldown	Ai-Chi			

DEEP-WATER DANCING 50-MINUTE WORKOUT

For most people, the difficulty here is to stay vertical and to remain in the same position in the water, but once you've mastered these problems, this is sure to become a favorite workout. To help keep you upright in the water, visualize a plumbline attached to your big toes, pulling them down to the pool floor. Another trick is to keep your abdominals contracted and your back relaxed. Once you've gained control, you'll be able to keep your trunk vertical in the water. To help you stay in the same position in the water, choose three visual reference points: one above you, one in front, and one beside you. Try to remain in the same position with respect to these three points by using your hands to contrast the movements of your legs.

Exercise	Mins	Objective	Muscle Groups	Intensity	Page
Warmup	8–10	Preparatory	All	Rhythmic limbering & static stretching	
Octopus 1	3	Aerobic	Quads, hamstrings	Moderate	72
Octopus 2	3	Aerobic	Quads, hamstrings	Moderate	74
Octopus 1 & 2	4	Aerobic	Quads, hamstrings	Moderate	
Octopus 3	3	Aerobic	Quads, hamstrings	Moderate	76
Octopus 1, 2, & 3	4	Aerobic	Quads, hamstrings	Moderate	
Octopus 4	3	Aerobic	Quads, hamstrings, hip mobility	Moderate	78
Octopus 1, 2, 3 & 4	4	Aerobic	Quads, hamstrings, hip mobility	Moderate	
Octopus 5	3	Aereobic	Quads, hamstrings, glutes, adductors	Moderate	80
Octopus 1, 2, 3, 4 & 5	4	Aerobic	Quads, hamstrings glutes, adductors	Moderate	
Jumping Jack Combination	3	Aerobic	Abductors, adductors	Moderate	44
Stride Combination	1	Aerobic	Glutes, iliopsoas	Moderate	82
One Leg Kick to Turn Combination	5	Aerobic	Glutes, iliopsoas	High	84
High Kick Combination	5	Aerobic	Glutes, iliopsoas	High	88
Cooldown	5	Stretching & relaxation	All	Low	

DEEP-WATER SPORT-CIRCUIT TRAINING PROGRAM 50-MINUTE WORKOUT

Here is a fun, deep-water workout where you can pace yourself according to your personal fitness level and objectives. With easy, repetitive moves, the aim is to work out as hard as you can in a full range of motion, while trying to maintain perfect alignment. Although not listed below, the abdominal muscles will work constantly to stabilize the body in a vertical position — keeping the upper body still during aerobic phases, and keeping the legs extended down to the floor during the upper body muscle-conditioning moves. If holding the vertical position causes stress on the back, pull your knees up to your chest.

Exercise	Mins	Objective	Muscle Groups	Intensity	Page
Warmup	8–10	Preparatory	All	Rhythmic limbering & static stretching	
Deep-water Jogs	3	Aerobic	Quads, hamstrings	Moderate to high	42
Bilateral Pullbacks	3	Muscle-conditioning	Traps, posterior delts	High	94
Deep-water Cycling	3	Aerobic	Quads, hamstrings	Moderate to high	106
Bilateral Crossovers	3	Muscle-conditioning	Pecs, anterior delts	High	94
Deep-water Gazelles	3	Aerobic	Glutes, iliopsoas	Moderate to high	104
Bilateral Pressbacks	3	Muscle-conditioning	Lats	High	96
Deep-water Jogs	3	Aerobic	Quads, hamstrings	Moderate to high	106
Triceps Kickbacks	3	Muscle-conditioning	Triceps, traps	High	92; 94
Deep-water Cycling	3	Aerobic	Quads, hamstrings	Moderate to high	106
Floating Reverse Curls	3	Muscle-conditioning	Rectus abdominus	High	98
Deep-water Gazelles	3	Aerobic	Quads, hamstrings	Moderate to high	49
Floating Lower Body Twist	3	Muscle-conditioning	Abs	High	48
Cooldown	5	Relaxation & stretching	All		

SPECIAL POPULATIONS

Aquafitness is an exercise modality suitable for most healthy people. Some groups, however, may need to adapt exercises to their specific conditions. These "special populations" include perinatal, children, obese, and seniors. Special classes can be designed for these groups or they can be mainstreamed into regular classes. If you join a class, let your instructor know if you have any medical conditions or injuries, or any other personal information that requires consideration. If you are working on your own, the following advice may be helpful. Whatever the group or their needs, everybody should have fun with aquafitness.

Perinatal

This group includes pregnant women and women who have given birth within the last six weeks or who are still breastfeeding. They should:
• work out within their comfort zone.
• use perceived exertion to determine the optimum intensity rate.
• drink plenty of water before, during, and after exercise.
• not overstretch the joints. A hormone that is released during the first trimester of pregnancy relaxes the joints, rendering them unstable.
• avoid any exercise or condition that could be dangerous for mother or baby.

Children

This group can be subdivided according to age and motor-skill development, but on the whole, kids just want to have fun. They should:
• work out within their comfort zones.
• use perceived exertion to determine the intensity rate.
• drink plenty of water before, during, and after exercise.
• do interval or circuit training workouts, changing the exercises often to hold their attention.
• include different levels of difficulty.
• be given lots of positive feedback.

Seniors

This group can benefit greatly from exercising in water. To ensure a safe and effective workout, they should:
• work out within their comfort zones.
• use perceived exertion to determine the intensity rate.
• drink plenty of water before, during, and after exercise.
• do aquatic strength training and muscle conditioning.
• include flexibility and range of motion exercises.
• keep the program activity simple.
• make the workout an enjoyable social event as well.

Overweight / obese

For many overweight people, water is the only exercise environment possible. These exercisers should:
• work out within their comfort zones.
• use perceived exertion to determine the intensity rate.
• drink plenty of water before, during, and after exercise.
• alternate weight-bearing and non-weight-bearing exercise (shallow and deep water).
• perform a full range of motion exercises.
• keep the exercises simple.

Aquafitness is safe for almost everybody, with very few exceptions. The important thing is to adapt your workout to your needs and objectives.

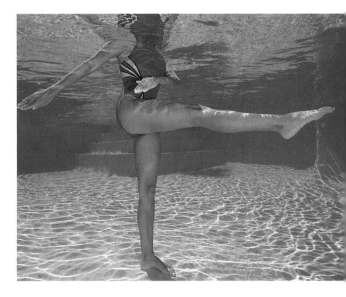

GLOSSARY

Abduction
movement away from the midline of the body
Adduction
movement towards the midline of the body
Aerobic
exercise requiring the supply of oxygen to the
muscles via the cardiorespiratory system
Agonist
the muscle of a pair that contracts actively at any
given time; also called the prime mover
Anaerobic
any activity performed in the absence of a quantity
of oxygen sufficient to avoid the accumulation of
lactic acid (fatigue) in muscle tissue
Anatomic position
the erect position of the body with all joints in their
natural positions; palms face the front
Antagonist
the muscle of a pair that relaxes or stretches
while the other muscle in the pair (the agonist)
contracts
Circumduction
circular movement at a joint (eg arm circles)
Extension
the increase of the angle formed between two
bones at the joint
External
outer, more superficial, closer to the skin
External rotation
rotating or turning a limb outwards
Flexion
the reduction of the angle formed between two
bones at the joint
Frontal plane
an imaginary plane that passes vertically through
the body and divides it in half, front and back
Horizontal abduction
moving the limb away from the midline of the
body horizontally
Horizontal adduction
moving the limb towards the midline of the
body horizontally
Hyperextension
moving a joint past the anatomical position
Internal
inner, deeper, closer to the centre of the body
Internal rotation
rotating or turning the limb inwards

Lactic acid
the byproduct of anaerobic glycolysis, which causes a
burning sensation in the muscle and results in
muscle fatigue – to be avoided in aerobic exercise
Lateral
away from the centre or midline of the body
Ligament
a tough fibrous band that connects bone to bone
Medial
towards the centre or midline of the body
Midline
imaginary line that passes vertically through the
centre of the body from the head down
Muscle pair
two muscles that are usually located on opposite
sides of a joint and work together to produce and
control movement
Neutral position
position of the spine in which the four physiological
curves – cervical, thoracic, lumbar, and sacral – are
maintained
Pronation
turning the arms so the palms face downwards
Prone
lying face down
Repetition
one complete execution of an exercise or movement;
set number of moves performed without pausing
Rotation
the movement of a body part along its longitudinal
axis (eg twisting)
Sagittal plane
an imaginary plane that passes vertically through the
body and divides it in half, right and left
Set
number of movement repetitions performed
in a sequence
Supination
turning the arms so the palms face upwards
Supine
lying face up
Synergist
muscle that assists the agonist in performing its task
Tendon
a fibrous band that connects muscle to bone
Transverse plane
an imaginary plane that passes horizontally through
the body and divides it in half, upper and lower

USEFUL ADDRESSES

AQUAFITNESS ORGANIZATIONS

H_2O_z
Australian Organisation for Aquafitness Leaders
www.midcoast.com.au

For information on Ai Chi
Aquatic Therapy and Rehabilitation Institute (ATRI)
email: atri@up.net
www.atri.org

For information on Watsu®
Worldwide Aquatic Bodyworks Association (WABA)
email: info@waba.edu
www.waba.edu

Speedo Australia
100 Mileham Street
South Windsor
NSW 2756
Telephone: 02-4577-1688
www.speedo.com

Splash International
email: splash@crosslink.net
www.splashinternational.com

EQUIPMENT AND CLOTHING

The following companies manufacture and supply
specialist clothing and equipment for aquafitness,
including buoyancy and flotation aids and chlorine-
resistant swimwear.

Aqua Shop
email: aquashop@aquashop.com.au
www.aquashop.com.au

Aussie Step
email: aquamat@ozemail.com.au
www.aquamat.com

Ragalluf Swimwear
email: lorelle@au.gateway.net
www.ragalluf.webcentral.com.au

Ryall's Aquatic Equipment
email: ryallsbelts@optushome.com.au
www.ryallsbelts.com.au

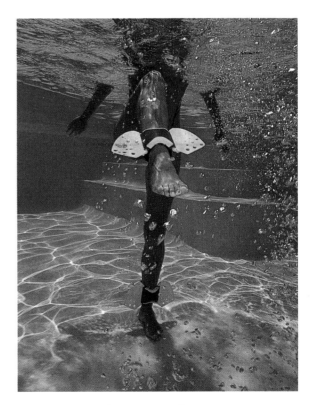

Once you've perfected your technique, equipment can
help you to continue improving your fitness level. Whatever you choose, buy the best quality you can afford.

INDEX

ACKNOWLEDGMENTS

Author's acknowledgments

I would like to give special thanks to:

My mother, Gladys Gonzalez Rodriguez, for always believing in me no matter what I do; my son, Paolo Emilio, for his active support and esteem; my husband, Paolo, for keeping his complaints within the norm; my mother-in-law, Pina Peja Adami, for her prayers.

Ludwig Artzt of Theraband GmbH and Herm Rottinghaus of Hygenic, Inc. for their continued support and use of their wonderful fitness products; Piscina Aventino in Rome for being a marvelous place to work, and all my wonderful clients, for their patience and inspiration as guinea pigs; everyone at SIAF (Scuola Italiana Aerobica e Fitness) for their support in putting up with my absences; everyone in the AEA (Aquatic Exercise Association) family for helping me grow in all aspects of aquafitness.

Terri Mitchell, for her friendship, comfort, and support always; June Lindle for her suggestions, invaluable information, and encouragement; Jun Konno and Ruth Sova, for the miracle that is Ai Chi; Danilo Vedruccio, Linda De Lehman, and Harold Dull for the inspiration that is Watsu®.

Pedro Franco, a dear friend and aquatic brother, you are with us always in every workout we'll ever do. Your work will continue.

Jenny Jones for a wonderful idea; Tracy Killick for a wild new vocabulary; Irene Lyford for her incredible patience and practical knowhow; Miranda Harvey for her artistic capabilities; and everyone at DK for their support and belief in aquafitness.

Zena Holloway, the photographer, and Ness, her assistant, for a wonderful job in not always easy conditions; all the models for being so professional and easy to work with: Hayley, Cathy, Russell, and Adele.

Aka, my cat, for keeping me company at all hours.

Publisher's acknowledgments

Dorling Kindersley would like to thank photographer Zena Holloway and her assistant Vanessa Sherry; models Hayley Yon, Cathy Ward, Russell Loom, and Adele Scholtz. We should also like to thank Annatjie Goedhals for her help in model casting in Cape Town; and Gavin at 360° Productions in Cape Town.

Finally, Dorling Kindersley would like to thank Hilary Bird for compiling the Index.

About the author

MIMI ROGRUIGEZ ADAMI has a passion for water, music, and movement. She is a combination of cultures and life experiences, which culminate in her love of teaching. Uniting her professional expertise with her charisma, she is in great demand worldwide as a fitness lecturer. A New Yorker of Dominican heritage, Mimi moved to Rome, Italy, for love, and since 1987, directs SIAF, the Italian Aerobic and Fitness School, creating land and aquatic instructor training programs. In 2000, Mimi was invited to teach Fitness at Rome's Tor Vergata University. Mimi and her husband, Paolo Adami, live in Rome with their son, Paolo Emilio, and Aka, the water-loving cat.

About the photographer

ZENA HOLLOWAY's underwater career began at the age of 18, when she qualified as a PADI diving instructor. Specializing in underwater photography, Zena's unique style grew out of assisting film crews on underwater film shoots and commercials. Recent commissions have included shooting large Blue and Mako sharks off Martha's Vineyard, in the US, and photographing Octopus Spear fisherman in Zanzibar. Zena lives in west London with her partner and baby daughter. www.zenaholloway.com; represented by The Peter Bailey Company, Tel: +44 (0) 20 7935 2626, Fax: +44 (0) 20 7935 7557, www.peterbailey.co.uk